On Snake-Poison
Its Action And Its Antidote

by

A. Mueller

On Snake-Poison
Its Action and Its Antidote
by A. Mueller

ISBN: 978-93-64282-55-0

Published by

DOUBLE 9 BOOKS
2/13-B, Ansari Road
Daryaganj, New Delhi – 110002
info@double9books.com
www.double9books.com
Tel. 011-40042856

ABOUT THE AUTHOR

A. Mueller was a great author, he was very famous for his style of writing, the characterization he used to put in his book, novel etc. He got recognition for his work, his novel was very famous in earlies. His research used to cover Mueller's research covers various venomous snake species, examining the specific compositions of their venoms and the diverse ways in which these toxins affect the human body this book was based on on snake –poison, its action and its antidote. Each authors develops a unique voice and style, characterized by their use of language, narrative techniques, and thematic focuses. Some may favor concise, straightforward prose, while others prefer elaborate, descriptive language. His impact as an author on literature and culture can be significant. Influential authors shape literary movements, inspire future writers, and leave a lasting mark on their readers.

CONTENTS

PREFACE

Since the method of treating snakebite-poisoning by hypodermic injections of strychnine, discovered by the writer and published but a few years ago, has already been adopted by the medical profession throughout the Australian colonies, and practised even by laymen in cases of urgency with much success, it has been repeatedly suggested to him that the subject calls for further elucidation at his hands; that the morbid processes engendered by the snake venom and the *modus operandi* of the antidote should be explained by him in a manner satisfying the demands of science, and at the same time within the grasp of the intelligent, moderately educated layman. When the latter, in a case of pressing emergency and in the absence of medical aid, is called upon to administer a potent drug in heroic doses, the aggregate of which would be attended by serious consequences in the absence of the deadly ophidian virus, an intelligent insight alone into the process he is about to initiate will give him that decision and promptitude of action, on the full exercise of which on his part it may depend whether, within a few hours, a valuable and to him probably dear life will be saved or lost.

The foregoing applies, not to Australia only, but to all other countries infested by venomous snakes. The introduction of the writer's method in every one of these countries is merely a question of time, for snake-poison acts everywhere according to one uniform principle, however different the symptoms it produces may appear to the superficial observer. The antidote, therefore, that cures snakebite in Australia will as surely cure it elsewhere if properly and efficiently applied.

To his Australian confrères, more especially to those who adopted his method but had to practise it more or less empirically, the writer also owes a more elaborate explanation of his theory of the action of snake-poison in all its bearings on the various nerve centres than is to be found in the scattered writings he has from time to time published in our periodical literature. His warmest thanks are due to them for the records of cases they have furnished to the *Australasian Medical Gazette*, and to the Hon. J. M. Creed, its able editor, for the ample space he has invariably allotted to the subject, and the valuable support he has given him throughout. By our united efforts we have reared in a dark and hitherto barren field of research a column of solid knowledge, and on this column Australia now occupies the highest and will ever occupy the most prominent place.

Not the least pleasing feature in the history of this discovery is the fact that it has been made without an elaborate series of experiments on animals, that it is a peaceful conquest not attained by means of doubtful justification, and which have hitherto invariably failed in their object. This object—the discovery of the coveted antidote—instead of being brought nearer, was, in fact, further removed by every succeeding series of experiments. However fruitful in results this mode of research has been in other domains, in this particular one it has not only been a failure but an actual bar to progress. Nature invariably refused to yield her secret when thus interrogated. The tortured animals, like the victims of Torquemada, either did not answer at all or they answered with a lie, and the baffled experimenter abandoned his task in despair.

Still, these negative results notwithstanding, the writer is confronted by a certain class of would-be rigorous scientists, who tell him that his theory of the action of snake-poison, though it explains all the phenomena, cannot be accepted as correct until it has been proven so by strict test experiments on animals, and that the successful administration of the antidote is proof only of the fact of neither antidote nor snake-poison having killed the patients, who, probably, might have recovered if left to themselves. This may be strict logic, but common sense replies to it that if recovery takes place after proper administration of the antidote in cases which, according to all our previous experience, would have ended fatally, it is not illogical to assume that antidote and recovery stand in the relation of cause and effect. This sceptical attitude of the scientific mind can justly be maintained only with regard to cases limited in number and in which the symptoms left room for doubt as to their final result, but in view of the formidable and constantly increasing records of cures from snakebite during the last three years, it is, to say the least of it, unreasonable.

The demand for experiments on animals, in proof of the correctness of his theory, the writer does not feel called upon to satisfy, for, apart from the theory proving itself by explaining all the symptoms the snake-poison produces, it has also stood the test of practical application. It is proven to be correct by the success of the antidote to which it led, and which is the logical outcome of it. After finally attaining a goal one has striven for, it is quite unnecessary to retrace one's steps with a view of ascertaining whether the road that has led up to it is the right and proper one.

By a fortuitous concurrence of circumstances, however, even this demand for experiments shall be satisfied in these pages. The writer published his theory of the action of snake-poison in May, 1888, after having practised the strychnine treatment for some years and thoroughly satisfied himself of its efficacy. In the latter part of 1888 accounts of Feoktistow's researches reached this country. His final conclusions to the effect that snake-poison is solely a nerve poison, that it does not destroy protoplasm, and has no effect whatever on the blood to which its destructive potency on animal life can be ascribed, were in complete harmony with the writer's views, in fact, a re-statement of his theory. It was a strange coincidence, or whatever it may be called, that, independent of each other, at almost opposite parts of the globe, and by opposite methods, we had arrived at almost identical conclusions. Those of Feoktistow were drawn from 400 elaborate experiments on animals, both vertebrates and invertebrates, made in the laboratory of Professor Kobert at the University of Dorpat and in that of Professor Owsjannikow at the Imperial Academy of Sciences of St. Petersburg. The writer's conclusions, on the other hand, resulted entirely from a careful and happy analysis of the symptoms observed at the bedside of his patients suffering from snakebite. On one point only, but the most important one, he differs from Feoktistow. The latter shared the fate of all previous experimenters on animals. Though his experiments with snake-poison led him to the correct theory of its action, and even to the correct antidote, his experiments with strychnine and snake-poison were a failure. The animals experimented on died, and, falling into the error of his predecessors, mistaking the functional analogy that exists between the nerve centres of the lower animals and those of man for absolute identity, which does not exist, especially not when they are under the influence of the two poisons, he concluded his researches with the confession that a physiological antidote for snake-poison cannot even be thought of at the present state of science. Although, therefore, Feoktistow's labors would have led to no practical result, they are, nevertheless, a most valuable contribution to science as being the first to demonstrate the action of snake-poison on a strictly scientific, experimental basis. For this reason, and with so high an authority as Professor Kobert vouching for the correctness of the experiments, they will be frequently quoted hereafter.

HISTORICAL REVIEW

Snakebite and its cure have always been the despair of medical science. On no other subject has our knowledge remained for centuries so unsatisfactory, fragmentary and empirical. The history of the subject, in fact, may be summed up briefly as a series of vain and spasmodic attempts to solve the problem of snakebite-poisoning and wring from nature the coveted antidote.

Various and contradictory theories of the action of snake-poison have been propounded, some absolutely erroneous, others containing a modicum of truth mixed with a large proportion of error, but none but one fulfilling the indispensable condition of accounting for all the phenomena observable during the poisoning process and of reducing the formidable array of conflicting symptoms to order by finding the law that governs them all. We have the advocates of the blood-poison theory ascribing the palpable nerve-symptoms to imaginary blood changes produced by the subtle poison, and alleged to have been discovered by the willing, but frequently deceiving microscope. Even bacteriology has been laid under service and innocent leucocytes have been converted under the microscope into deadly germs, introduced by the reptile, multiplying with marvellous rapidity in the blood of its victims, appropriating to themselves all the available oxygen and producing carbonic acid, as the saccharomyces does in alcoholic fermentation. Others again, and among them those supposed to be the highest authorities on the subject now living, divide the honors between nerve and blood. Some snakes they allege are nerve-poisoners others as surely poison the blood, but with one solitary exception they assume the terminations of the motor-nerves and not the centres to be affected.

Thus then with regard to theories we have hitherto had "confusion worse confounded," and as with theories so it has been with antidotes. They were proposed in numbers, but only to be given up again, some intended to decompose and destroy the subtle poison in the system, others to counteract its action on the system with that action unknown. It is scarcely too much to assert that there are but few chemicals and drugs in the materia medica that have not been tried as antidotes in experiments on animals and dozens upon dozens that have been tried in vain on man.

The reasons for this somewhat chaotic state of our science on a subject of so much interest to mankind are various. The countries of Europe, in which scientific research is most keenly pursued, have but few indigenous, and these comparatively harmless snakes. The best scientific talent has, therefore, only exceptionally been brought to bear on the subject. In those countries on the other hand in which venomous snakes abound and opportunities for observing the poison-symptoms on man are more plentiful, the observing element has been comparatively deficient.

A still more potent source of failure must be sought in the faulty methods of research pursued by most investigators. Experiments on animals were far too much resorted to, and their frequently misleading results accepted as final, whilst observations on man did not receive the attention their importance demanded.

In the investigation of this subject the first desideratum was no doubt to find the correct theory of the action of snake poison and to define the law governing that action, assuming as a working hypothesis that there is but one law for all snake-poison and not several ones, just as there is one law for the structure of these reptiles, admitting of variations, but not of absolute divergence from the general plan. The shortest and surest way to find this law is close observation and careful analysis of the symptoms produced by the poison on man, and as the opportunities for such observation are not of frequent occurrence to the individual, co-operation and careful comparison of notes on the part of many observers.

This method of investigation, which, during the last few years, has been pursued in Australia with most satisfactory results, was never practised anywhere else, not even in America, but instead of it each observer, with few exceptions, kept his own notes to himself, and if there happened to be one here and there hungry for more knowledge than his scanty opportunities for observation on man would supply, his resort was usually experiments on animals. A few snakes were caught, a few luckless dogs or other animals procured, and the slaughter of the innocents began.

As test experiments to confirm observations on man, or made with a view of finding a correct theory of the action of snake-poison, these attempts were unobjectionable, although, without an elaborate scientific apparatus and in other than skilled hands, they were not likely to produce results of any value. But most of the experimenters were not content with purely theoretical aims. They were seeking to find the antidote by a purely empirical method, and had nothing to guide them in the choice of drugs. A dose of snake-poison was administered to an animal, and then a dose of some drug or chemical, chosen *ad libitum*, sent after it. Next day another presumed antidote was tried, another animal slaughtered, and so on *ad nauseam*, until finally the baffled antidote-searcher, not one whit the wiser for all his trouble and the useless tortures inflicted, confessed himself beaten and joined in the *"non possums"* of his predecessors.

One important point has been completely left out of sight and ignored in all this experimenting on animals. It is the fact that the action of snake-poison on the human system and on that of animals, more especially dogs, though very similar, is not absolutely identical, and that for this reason alone results of experiments on the latter cannot be indiscriminately applied to man. As pointed out before, analogy has been confounded with identity. When a dog, for instance, has been bitten by a snake he does not usually collapse as quickly as a human being, but is able to drag himself about much longer before his hind legs refuse their service and he is unable to walk. This longer duration of the first stage of the poisoning process is no doubt owing to a higher organisation and greater functional power of the motor nerve centres of dogs. The amount of motor force at their disposal is greater, and hence they offer greater resistance to the invader seeking to turn off this force. When finally the latter gains the ascendency, irregular discharges of motor nerve force still take place and find their expression in convulsions, which in man only exceptionally occur. But the difference between man and dog becomes more marked yet when strychnine is administered to a dog suffering from snake-poison. It counteracts the latter quite as effectually in a dog as in man, but has to be injected with extreme caution, for whilst in man a slight excess in the quantity required to subdue the snake-virus is not only harmless, but actually necessary, any excess of it in a dog will at once produce violent tetanic convulsions and cause the animal to die even quicker than the snake-poison would have killed it, if allowed to run its course. In the face of these facts the judiciousness of the proposal lately made both here and in India to subject the strychnine treatment of snakebite once more to a series of test experiments on animals appears more than questionable.

Another cause that has largely contributed to render experiments on animals so barren of results must be sought in the injudicious selection of substances intended to serve as antidotes. It is simply impossible to act on an organic compound like snake-poison, coursing through a living system, by chemicals that will either combine with it or decompose it in a manner likely to deprive it of its deadly qualities and render it innocuous. Yet what do we find? Acids and alkalis, arsenic, bromides and iodides, chlorine, mercurial preparations, &c., &c., have been poured into the luckless animals as if they were so many test tubes. A chemical antidote, a substance possessing special affinity to snake-poison and by means of this affinity combining with it in some mysterious and incomprehensible manner, one can hardy imagine to exist. Physiological antidotes, on the other hand, substances acting on the system in a manner the exact reverse of, and in direct antagonism to the snake-poison, though apparently the only feasible ones, have been strangely neglected and almost despised by experimenters.

In the vast storehouse of Nature the department most likely to furnish such antidotes is the vegetable kingdom. The untutored human mind has for centuries past intuitively clung to this idea, and sought among plants for remedies against the deadly ophidian poison. Hence the great number of vegetable antidotes that have from time to time been recommended and the efficacy of some of which at least has been confirmed by reliable observations. But the hint thus given to science was not taken. Instead of research being pushed on diligently in the only direction that promised any chance of success, it was cut short by the baneful method of experimenting on animals. When it had been demonstrated that a dog, a cat, or other animal, after having been saturated with snake-poison, did not recover after the administration of an alleged antidote, the illogical conclusion was drawn at once that it could not possibly be of any use to man, whilst, in reality, the only proof rendered by the experiment, if made properly, was that the respective antidote could not be relied on in treating animals of the class experimented on. That some of these despised antidotes are worth a little further investigation may, in the light of present experience as to the value of strychnine in snakebite, be inferred from the fact, that among them is the wood of *Strychnos Colubrina*, and also the well-known *Huang Noo*, a vegetable extract made from another variety of the Strychnos family, and largely used by the Chinese, whilst, according to a letter in the *Australasian Medical Gazette*, July, 1892, the principal ingredient of a strange compound used by the native snake doctors of Central America with much success is *Nux Vomica*.

It is superfluous to enter into a criticism of the treatment of snakebite until recently in vogue, for, with the exception of the local one by ligature and excision, it stands self-condemned by its complete inefficiency. It may be summed up as a vain attempt to stem the collapse invariably attending snakebite by the administration of stimulants, such as alcohol, ether, ammonia, &c. The attempt is vain, for a person in collapse from snakebite cannot be stimulated by any of these remedies, since neither the heart nor the nerve centres respond to them in the slightest degree, as they do in the absence of snake-poison, the only one that has any effect at all in slight cases being ammonia. But the attempt is not only in vain, it is highly injurious, especially if made with the usual large doses of alcohol, for, in addition to the latter not having the slightest influence on the snake-poison and its baneful effects, they act as an anæsthetic and thus add to the existing depression, besides increasing the tendency to internal hæmorrhage.

It might, under these circumstances, have been expected that any new method of treating snakebite, based on scientific grounds and holding out a sure prospect of success, would be hailed with pleasure, and that conservatism, opposing the new simply on account of its newness, would refrain from its usual tactics in a case where there was really nothing to conserve. But this was not to be, and strange, indeed, it would have been if the writer had escaped the opposition which is almost invariably offered to the discoverer. It appears to be one of the laws of human evolution, wisely designed to prevent precipitate advance, that every new discovery must run the gauntlet of men whose mission it is to act as brakes on the wheels of progress. Of the opposition which has been offered to the strychnine treatment it would, therefore, be folly to complain, but just cause of complaint is furnished by the unscientific attitude which was assumed from the very first and has been maintained throughout by its opponents.

Not a single attempt has been made to disprove the correctness of the theory on which it is founded, yet to leave this theory unquestioned but object to the conclusion to which it leads, must strike even the lay mind as a most illogical proceeding. It is self-evident that, when strychnine is administered as an antidote to snake-poison, the quantity of it injected must be in proportion to that of snake-venom present in the system, and that the doses in which we dispense it in ordinary practice must be entirely left out of sight. Still, in the face of these obvious conclusions, we have had veterans, grave and grey, arguing pompously that the heroic doses advocated by the writer could not be countenanced, and that even medical men could not be entrusted with the serious task of administering them. Even as late as the last medical congress at Sydney this absurd objection to large doses of the antidote was again brought forward. After quantities averaging from half a grain to a grain have been injected many times in Australia with continuous success, after Banerjee has even gone as high as three and four grains in India without a single failure, and without in one single instance serious strychnine symptoms being evoked, the writer of the paper on "Snakebite and its Cure" based his principal objection to the treatment on the alleged ground of there not being sufficient evidence before us to justify heroic doses and show them to be safe in practice. When people wilfully shut their eyes against the most conclusive evidence, it is improbable that any amount of it would satisfy them. Apart, however, from the fully proven antagonism between the two poisons rendering the large doses of the antidote, which in all serious cases are indispensable, perfectly safe, the fear of strychnine is, in itself, a very strange aberration of judgment on the part of my opponents, considering how easy it is to counteract any noteworthy excess in its action, if, perchance, it should occur through unnecessary overdosing, by appropriate remedies.

All other objections to the treatment require but to be glanced at to show their absurdity. Certain crude experiments on dogs made many years ago in India, and put forward as irrefutable at first, have been abandoned of late, and my learned opponents have now taken up a position in their stronghold of statistics, supposed to be impregnable, but in reality only the last refuge of the destitute, a position from which, by dexterous handling of alleged facts, anything and everything can be proven, in short, to use a strong expression, not my own, a convenient and respectable form of lying. By means of these statistics they try to prove, in the first place, that Australian snake-poison is not at all the insidious death-dealing agent it is supposed to be, since, according to statistics, only 126 persons died from it in three colonies within the last ten years. Further study of these statistics leads them to the inference that a strong healthy adult will recover from snakebite *without any treatment*, and thus they finally arrive at the conclusion aimed at, that persons cured by strychnine injections would probably have recovered without them. These are the inferences drawn by men, who, practising in towns, have probably never seen a case of snakebite. How do they tally with the facts of the case? It is true that the mortality among those bitten by snakes is small here as compared with India, though the poison of our snakes, quantity for quantity, has been proven to be quite as deadly as that of the Indian ones. Our greater immunity is due to our snakes giving off less poison at a bite, and with their short and (excepting those of the death adder) merely grooved poison fangs injecting it very superficially, thus making the process of elimination of the poison by ligature and incision or excision of the punctures much more easy and successful. It is to this treatment, which, as a rule; is immediately adopted in the bush, that our small mortality is due. Our children are taught it in school, and the most illiterate bushman knows how to carry it out. Where it is omitted by persons not knowing that they are bitten until the poison has been absorbed recovery is as rare as it is with the ox and the horse left to themselves without any treatment. But it requires a prodigious stretch of the logical faculty to understand what our small mortality from snakebite has to do with the intrinsic merits of the strychnine treatment. Even if nobody died at all its effects in doing away with the misery and suffering, which, before its introduction, invariably followed snakebite, and often was never got rid of completely, would still be sufficiently beneficial to render the senseless opposition to it on the part of a small section of medical men little short of criminal; for these effects are a matter of constant observation, and cannot, like the rescues from death, be called into question.

The statistics brought forward to prove that the treatment has not reduced the death-rate are also most faulty. Until it is thoroughly understood and in every instance properly applied it is manifestly foolish as well as unfair to lay non-success and failures at its door. When a medical man is called upon to treat a serious case, and instead of boldly addressing himself to the task of combating the symptoms by injecting the antidote irrespective of the quantity he may require until it has conquered the snake-poison, becomes nervous and ceases to inject, when, after what in ordinary practice would be a dangerous dose, he sees but little effect, or if from the first he injects small doses at long intervals, the cause of failure surely lies with him and not with the antidote, which rarely fails where it is properly applied. The duty of disseminating a sound knowledge of the principles of the strychnine treatment unquestionably devolves on our health authorities, who ought, by this time, to have taken some notice of it. But officialdom remains obtuse and issues circulars on the treatment of snakebite, recommending, *inter alia,* the free use of alcohol.

The literature on the subject of snake-poison is very voluminous, but those who seek for enlightenment in it will be as disappointed as the writer was after wading through it. The toilers in this barren field of research were numerous, but with few exceptions, they toiled in vain. Fontana may be looked upon as the founder of that hideous experimentalism by which, in his hands alone, four thousand animals were tortured to death without a single tangible result except that in his great work, "Reserche Fisiche sopra il Veneno della Vipera," which he wrote at the conclusion of his cruel labours, he left us a grotesque monument of patient, but ill-guided research. Other Italians, following his method, Redi, Mangili, Metaxa, &c., were equally unsuccessful in shedding one ray of light on the vexed and obscure problem.

Among the Germans who contributed to the subject may be mentioned:—

Wagner.—"Erfahrungen über den Biss der gemeinen Otter."

Prinz Maximilian von Wiedd.—"Beiträge zur Geschichte Brasiliens."

Lenz.—"Schlangenkunde."

Heinzel.—"Ueber Pelias Berus und Vipera Ammodytes."

Among the French:—

Soubeiran.—"Rapport sur les Vipéres de France."

Bullet.—"Etude sur la Mosure de Vipére."

British and American Workers are the most numerous. Commencing with the century we have:—

Russell.—"An Account of Indian Serpents, collected on the Coast of Coromandel." Later on,

S. Weir Mitchell.—"Researches upon the Venom of the Rattlesnake."

Halford—"On Australian Snakes, and the Intravenous Injection of Ammonia, in *British Medical Journal*, *Medical Times*, and *Australian Medical Journal*."

Jones.—"On Trigonocephalus Contortrix."

Nicholson.—"On Indian Snakes."

Sir Joseph Fayrer.—"The Tanatophidia of India." Also, "Researches in conjunction with Richards, Brunton and Eward."

Wall.—"On the Difference in the Physiological Effects produced by the Poison of Indian Venomous Snakes." Proc. Royal Soc., 1881, vol. xxxii., p. 333.

Among those enumerated above Wall is the only one who formulated a correct and thoroughly scientific theory of the action of snake-poison, which has since been confirmed by Australian research and by Feoktistow's elaborate experiments. It is strange that, after finding the theory that explained all the phenomena, he did not follow it up by applying the antidote to which his theory should have led him.

SNAKE-POISON AND ITS ACTION

The poison gland of snakes is the analogue of the parotid gland of mammals, both in position and structure. Its acini or alveoli are lined with a layer of secretory, columnar, finely granular cells and arranged with great regularity along the excretory duct, which is straight and cylindrical and opens with vipers into the hollow poison fang, with our colubrines into the groove on the anterior surface of it. Snake-poison, as it leaves this gland, is a thin, albuminoid, yellow liquid of neutral reaction. On exposure to the air it becomes viscid and slightly acid. Of its chemical composition we know as yet but little, and it is very questionable whether the most perfect chemical analysis of its constituents would ever have given us a clue to its action or will enrich our present knowledge of it. Like all albuminoid secreta it becomes putrid after prolonged exposure and then, through ammonia production, loses its acid, and assumes an alkaline reaction, still, however, though in a modified degree, retaining its toxic properties, which are completely lost only after an exposure of many months. Feoktistow found that freezing at 1° R. caused the poison to separate into a solid mass and a thin, very yellow liquid, which, even at a temperature of 4° R., remained liquid, and the poisonous properties of which greatly exceeded those of the solid mass. Boiling diminishes and, continued for any length of time, completely destroys the potency of the poison.

The microscope has done good service in the investigation of snake-poison. It has, in the first place, informed us with absolute certainty that there are no micro-organisms or germs of any kind in the fresh poison immediately after it leaves the gland. But a still more important revelation we owe to it is the fact that these organisms, when we introduce them into a 2% solution of the poison, do not die, but live, multiply, and enjoy their existence most lustily, as they do in any other non-poisonous albuminoid liquid, whilst animals of a higher type—say a snail or a frog—soon perish in it. In watching the movements of the latter we find that they get slower and slower, and finally cease. We now follow up the interesting research, and take two frogs. Under the skin of one of them we inject a few drops of the poison solution, the other one for comparison we leave intact, and place both into a glass globe partly filled with water. In a very short time we have no difficulty to identify the poisoned frog. Its hind legs begin to drop and their movements become sluggish. This difficulty increases from minute to minute, until at last all motion ceases, and the legs hang down completely paralysed. At the same time we observe that the animal shows increasing difficulty of breathing, that, even when taken out of the water, and placed on the table before us it gasps for breath and is unable to move. At last respiration ceases altogether and the frog dies.

Two problems now present themselves for solution. In the first place we have to account for the fact of the snake-poison leaving the lower forms of animal life intact and being fatal to the higher ones. The symptoms we have observed in the frog point unmistakably to an affection of the nervous system as their cause. Now we know that the lower forms which the poison does not affect have no such system, and we are justified to infer that to the absence of this system they owe their immunity. This inference leads us on to a second one equally justifiable, namely, that there is a certain unaccountable attraction between the delicate nerve tissue and the subtle ophidian poison, which renders the latter a specific nerve poison.

Our second problem is to ascertain the nature of the change in the nerves, to find out, if possible, whether it is merely functional or an actual interference with the structure of either cells or fibres. With this end in view we once more consult the microscope. We make two preparations, one of nerve fibres and of nerve cells of the poisoned frog, and, under the microscope, compare them carefully with an analogous one from the killed healthy frog. The result is purely negative as regards structural change. Both present identical and perfectly normal pictures of apparently healthy cells and fibres. There being no visible structural change we are driven to the conclusion that only a functional one has been effected by the poison, and with the symptoms observed all pointing in that direction, that it is of central origin.

The writer's theory as to the action of snake-poison, formed, in the first instance from observations made at the bedside of his patients only, is thus confirmed by experiments specially instituted by him for that purpose. Further proof of its correctness we have in the brilliant results of the strychnine treatment of snakebite in Australia, which is the outcome and practical application of this theory. In those desperate cases more especially, reported from all parts of the colonies, in which death was imminent, and pulse at wrists as well as respiration had already ceased, the strychnine injections could not possibly have effected complete recovery within a few hours if the structure of the nerve centres had been impaired or blood changes brought about incompatible with life.

Feoktistow's experiments, made with viper poison, fully bear out the correctness of the writer's theory, besides proving that there is no essential difference between the action of the viperine and colubrine poisons. He proved conclusively that snake-poison does not destroy protoplasm or interfere with infusorial life, that injected into the heart of a mollusc it causes an almost immediate cessation of its action, that hypodermic injections of it in fish produce contraction of the pigment cells and bleaching of the integuments, followed by asphyxial respiration, general paralysis and death. Similar results were observed on frogs. In mammals the symptoms were: dyspnoea, asphyxia, paresis and paralysis of the lower extremities with succeeding general paralysis, sometimes tonic and clonic convulsions, hæmorrhages from bowels, lungs, nose and bladder, and finally complete paralysis of respiration and of heart.

Action of Snake-Poison on Special Nerve Centres

It must be borne in mind that the symptoms as about to be detailed are successive only to some extent in the order presented. They commence generally at the lower part of the spinal cord, but immediately afterwards, if not simultaneously, are ushered in with great rapidity from other centres, masking each other and rendering it extremely difficult to observe and analyse them separately. They are also very variable through the poison concentrating its action on special centres, leaving others comparatively intact, and this not only when from different varieties of snakes, but also from snakes of the same variety. Another element increasing the difficulties of correct analysis are the depressing effects of fear, inseparable in all but the strongest minds from the consciousness of having been bitten, and so similar in appearance to those of snake-poison, that sometimes it is by no means easy to decide which of the two is in operation, and that only those cases are of real value to the observer from which this element of fear is completely excluded.

A.—Action on the Anterior Cornua of the Spinal Cord

The anterior cornua are almost invariably the first of the motor-centres attacked by the snake-poison, the affection (commencing with paresis and in serious cases generally culminating in paralysis) beginning in the lumbar ganglia and taking an upward course. The lower extremities feel unnaturally heavy and a paretic condition of the muscles supervenes *simultaneously on both sides.* The walk becomes unsteady and staggering, very similar to that of persons under the influence of large doses of alcohol. By a powerful effort of the will, however, persons in this condition are often able to walk and even run for some distance, especially if by prompt ligature the absorption of the poison has been checked. As the affection proceeds, though still able to move the legs in a sitting posture, they are unable to rise again. Ere long even sitting up becomes impossible and they collapse helplessly. At this stage sensation is still intact, and reflex action, by pricking the skin, &c., still takes place. The upper extremities generally retain the power of voluntary motion, even after the muscles of the neck have become paretic and the head is held up with difficulty or sinks to one side.

With birds, according to Feoktistow, the reverse is the case. The wings are usually first attacked, or paresis comes on in wings and legs at the same time.

B.—Action on the Medulla Oblongata

a.—The Vaso-Motor Centre

Whilst the voluntary muscles are thus brought under the influence of the poison, symptoms denoting the invasion of the oblongata are rapidly developing. The first of these is the deadly pallor and ashy hue of the cold skin, evidently due to the blood receding from the surface, a condition not unlike that obtaining in extreme anæmia. As persons in this state complain of an agonising feeling about the heart and of deadly faintness, a paretic condition of the heart suggests itself as the most obvious cause, more especially when taken in conjunction with the small, frequent, and compressible pulse. But though the heart muscle is no doubt participating in the general paresis, the condition of the surface of the body is in reality one of anæmia. The blood, even at this early stage, begins to accumulate in the large veins of the abdomen, which expand gradually in consequence of the diminishing motor force supplied by the splanchnicus, keeping them in the normal state of contraction when intact and having its centre in the medulla oblongata. When this large vaso-motor nerve is cut in animals anywhere in its course, the veins of the abdomen become distended enormously. The animal is, so to say, bled into its own belly.

By a series of most interesting experiments Feoktistow has shown conclusively that snake-poison has the same effect on the abdominal circulation as section of the splanchnicus. Even slight intravenous injections of the poison produced quickly a high degree of paresis of the nerve and a corresponding engorgement of the veins of the abdomen, whilst after lethal doses, the paresis culminated in a few minutes in complete paralysis, followed by rapid collapse, excessive weakness of the bloodless heart, and death from paralysis of the latter and anæmia of the nerve-centres. One experiment deserves special record, as it also shows the untenability of the blood-poison theory.

The whole vascular system of an animal poisoned by intravenous injection was thoroughly washed out with the warm defibrinised blood of four animals of the same species, the blood being infused into an external jugular vein and allowed to flow out of a crural artery. Although blood exceeding its normal quantity was left in the animal, when the vessels named were closed, the nerve affection remained unchanged. The blood pressure raised during the infusion sank at once again to zero, when it ceased, and the paralysed veins of the abdomen became engorged once more with the whole, or nearly the whole, of the blood-mass, leaving the rest of the body anæmic as before. This interesting experiment also shows how strong a hold the snake-poison has on the nerve-cells when they are thoroughly under its influence, and how independent this paralysing action is of the blood, persisting, as it was in this case, after all the poison had been washed out of the animal.

The heart in vaso-motor paresis and paralysis is weakened in the first instance by the direct action of the poison on the medulla oblongata and the intracardiac ganglia. Its pulsations, at first retarded in frequency, become accelerated soon after the introduction of the poison, the pulse rate increasing rapidly and the waves becoming smaller and more easily compressible in proportion to the frequency of the pulse, which generally counts from 100 to 120 and more per minute at a comparatively early stage of the poisoning process. But an equally potent cause of heart failure is its depletion by the simultaneous stagnation of the blood mass in the veins of the abdomen. Finally, to complete the mischief, we have not only anæmia of the semi-paralytic oblongata, but the scanty blood supply this important centre receives becomes also surcharged with carbonic acid. Oxyhæmaglobin disappears almost entirely from the blood under the circumstances detailed, as both pulmonary and internal respiration are greatly interfered with, the blood tending more and more towards that thin dark condition which it presents after death, and which has been taken as *prima facie* evidence of the direct blood-poisoning action of snake virus by one and all of previous investigators.

That under the powerful combination of causes, each of which is in itself sufficient to endanger life, and greatly intensified as paresis gradually deepens into paralysis, the heart, even of large animals, succumbs in a comparatively short time, may be readily understood.

The *blood-pressure*, under the circumstances just detailed, must necessarily be *nil*. Observations by means of the sphygmograph at the bedside of a person suffering from snake-poison are scarcely feasible, except, perhaps, in a hospital, and thus far are not on record. We must, therefore, once more fall back on Feoktistow's experiments, which show that even the smallest doses (0.02 to 0.04 mllgr.) of the dried poison *per kilo* injected into the vein of a cat caused a fall in the blood-pressure almost immediately, without influencing either pulse or respiration, but that two to four mgr. were sufficient to reduce the blood-pressure to zero and bring on collapse, infusions of blood only raising it temporarily. Of drugs raising the blood-pressure he found ammonia the most effective, but only after slight doses of the poison; after lethal ones it had no effect whatever on the blood pressure but greatly increased the hæmorrhagic process in all internal organs. This important observation should be kept in mind by those who inject ammonia in serious snakebite cases, and it probably applies likewise to *the excessive use of alcohol*.

This leads the writer on to the discussion of this singular hæmorrhagic process principally characteristic of viperine poisoning, and only very exceptionally produced by the poison of colubrines. It is among the symptoms of snakebite poisoning one of the most interesting ones, but also one most difficult of explanation. There can be no doubt that it is produced by vaso-motor paresis and paralysis. We further know that it is preceded by dilatation of the capillaries and small veins, and that it is effected principally through the process known as diapedesis, or the passage of both red and white corpuscles with plasma through the unruptured capillary membrane, and even the thin one of small veins, which is nearly of the same structure, being composed of endothelial cells united by cement. This membrane possesses a certain degree of porosity, which is probably increased by dilatation. In the absence of plain muscular fibres contraction and dilatation of the capillaries can only be effected by a corresponding contraction and expansion of the nuclei of the endothelial cells. As fibrils derived from non-medullated nerves terminate in small end-butts in connection with the capillary membrane, we may assume that the nuclei of the endothelial cells are under the sway of vaso-motor nerve currents, that weak ones will expand, strong ones contract them. We may further assume that the red and white corpuscles force their way out of the vessels through pores in the cement substance, since a passage of cell through cell is not thinkable. Thus far we see our way fairly clear. But the question now arises: what causes the solid constituents of the blood to force their way through the capillary membranes all over the mucous surfaces, even the conjunctiva, and not these alone, but also through serous membranes such as the pericardium, and strangest of all, through old scars in the skin? If the most modern ideas as to the cause of diapedesis being blood pressure are correct, it is quite incomprehensible how it can take place in the absence of blood pressure, and take place so extensively. The theory of blood pressure may apply to diapedesis accompanying the inflammatory process. In snakebite poisoning it is more likely to be due to passive engorgement of the capillary system and probably also to blockage of corpuscles in the finest capillary tubes. In vaso-motor paresis, and still more paralysis, the arterioles supplying the capillaries are widely dilated, and at the lowest blood pressure probably send more blood into the latter than in the normal state. This circumstance in itself is apt to cause capillary engorgement. In the finest capillaries permitting only a string of corpuscles, one behind the other but none abreast, to pass through in the normal state, dilatation may cause blockage by two or three becoming wedged in abreast and closing the lumen of the vessel by a sort of embolism. On the arterial side of this obstruction the crowded corpuscles force their way through the porous cement substance by what little "vis a tergo" there may be left yet, whilst in the venous side, in the small veins corresponding with the closed capillaries, engorgement must necessarily take place through this "vis a tergo" being entirely absent, and diapedesis, which here also has been observed, follow in due course. The writer has always been inclined to take this view, the correctness of which appears to be borne out by an experiment recorded by Feoktistow. He found on sprinkling a two per cent. solution of snake-poison over the mesentery of an healthy animal, that wherever a drop of the solution fell, almost immediately the capillaries and small veins became dilated and small point-like effusions of blood appeared, gradually enlarging and ultimately becoming confluent with adjoining ones. Large hæmorrhagic surfaces were thus formed in a comparatively short time. Here paralysis of the nerve-cells interspersed in the vaso-motor nerve-ends was evidently the first effect, followed by dilatation of the capillaries and immediately afterwards by effusion. Without some obstruction within the capillaries, like that above described, effusion in this purely local poisoning process appears unexplainable.

The special preference which the viper-poison has for the vaso-motor sphere will hereafter be referred to. Hæmorrhages from Australian snake-poison are comparatively rare. Even at the bitten place there is as a rule very little swelling and effusion and frequently none at all. When it occurs it quickly disappears after strychnine injections. Only a few cases have been reported as yet of blood-vomiting. In one of these the hæmorrhage took place soon after the bite and was so considerable that it must have arisen from actual rupture of vessels consequent on abdominal engorgement and not from mere diapedesis. It is very doubtful whether the latter ever takes place here as it does after viper-bite in India and elsewhere. Even the death-adder, although half a viper, and producing more swelling and effusion locally than any other one of our snakes, is not known to have ever produced the extensive effusions from mucous surfaces in pericardium, lungs, &c., described above. More research however is necessary, especially more carefully conducted autopsies. Since Australia has taken the lead in this hitherto so obscure department, every practitioner should make it his object and special ambition to contribute his quota towards the elucidation of the subject, not only by reporting successful cases, but also the post-mortem appearances in unsuccessful ones, wherever it is practicable. It is not by experiments on animals but by a hearty co-operation of Australian practitioners that we can ever hope to supplement our knowledge on this subject.

b.—The Respiratory Centre

Paresis of this centre does not play as important a part here as it does in India, more especially after cobra-bite. The peculiar, and as yet unexplained, tendency of snake-poison to act with special virulence on some centres, passing others by comparatively little disturbed, is markedly shown by the cobra poison of India as compared with that of our Australian cobra (*hoplocephalus curtus.*) The unfortunate victims of the former are tortured by an ever-increasing dyspnoca, and finally die from asphyxia, under what are supposed to be carbonic acid convulsions. They retain their consciousness more or less unclouded to the last, the poison spending all its force on the respiratory centre, and leaving the brain intact. Here we hardly ever see actual dyspnoca after the bite of hoplocephalus or any other Australian snake. Respiration becomes quicker at an early stage, and then, from hour to hour, shallower; but our patients soon pass from sleep into coma, and suffer no respiratory distress even when, in consequence of general paralysis, the respiratory muscles cease to act, which usually takes place a few minutes before the heart stands still.

Feoktistow records the following observations on cats with reference to the respiratory centre:—Small intravenous injections of the fresh poison (0.07-0.13 mllgr.) produced a great increase in frequency of respirations (280-360 per minute). Section of both vagi at once reduced this frequency, from which he infers that small doses act as an irritant to the respiratory centre. When small doses were repeated several times, the respiratory movements were gradually retarded, and asphyxia set in through paralysis of the centre. Large doses produced this effect at once, without any previous acceleration. Very large ones paralysed respiration, heart, and vaso-motors almost simultaneously, and caused the blood pressure to fall to 0. By the kymograph respirations were found to become shallower in proportion to their frequency. As the latter was reduced, they became at first deeper, but ere long shallower again, and were occasionally interrupted by spasmodic inspirations. Artificial respiration prolonged life for a short time only.

C.—Action on Centres of Cranial Nerves

Among the symptoms denoting paresis of motor-centres of cranial nerves, together with sympathetic ganglia, the first and most noteworthy is the early dilatation of the pupil. This truly pathognomic condition is never absent, and becomes intense when paresis becomes intensified into paralysis. The most glaring light, in immediate proximity to the eyeball, has then no effect whatever on the pupil. If it remains dilated after strychnine injections have restored consciousness and the power to walk, it is a sure sign that the snake-poison is not completely counteracted, and will in all probability re-assert itself, necessitating another injection, whilst a pupil restored to its normal condition justifies the conclusion that the patient is safe.

Another symptom denoting paresis of the cranial nerve-centres is a marked change in the expression of the face. The features become relaxed, and lose their mimetic play. The cornea is dull, and, together with the anterior surface of the eyeball, becomes dry, as the eyelids are moved imperfectly, if at all, and the tears in consequence are not properly distributed over the conjunctiva. The nostrils become more or less immovable, and the naso-labial fold is obliterated, whilst the lower lip hangs down. The lips are apart, as the lower jaw is not held up by the muscles. When paralysis supervenes it drops entirely, and the tongue protrudes.

Deglutition, somewhat difficult in paresis, is completely suspended in the paralytic stage, through paralysis of the soft palate, the pharynx, and œsophagus. Liquids forced on the patient in this extremity may partly flow down the œsophagus, but will also enter the larynx, and their administration should be carefully avoided.

D. Action on motor-centres of Cerebellum and Basal Ganglia

Of this action little if anything is patent to observation. A certain want of co-ordination in the movements has been noticed in the early stage of paresis, and the peculiar staggering walk of persons in this stage is probably owing to an affection of the motor-centres of the cerebellum. That they do not escape the action of the subtle poison, when symptoms denoting the invasion of all the other motor-centres throughout the body are in evidence, we have every reason to assume. The co-ordination and automatic regulation of the lower motor-centres must necessarily escape observation when the function of these centres is partially suspended, and when, moreover, the powerful currents of nerve force the cerebellum and basal ganglia receive from the motor cortical centres of the cerebrum are partially if not wholly withdrawn.

E. Action of the Motor Cortical Centres of the Cerebrum

In all but the very lightest cases of snakebite-poisoning there are always symptoms manifested that cannot be referred to any other cause than an invasion of the centres now under consideration. They range from mere stupor, confusion of thought and delirium to the deepest coma, with complete extinction of consciousness and insensibility to all external impressions. Coma is a frequent and in serious cases an almost invariable symptom in Australia. After the bite of our death adder only we find persons sometimes collapse and expire suddenly, when still conscious and able to answer questions rationally. Coma invariably develops from sleep. It is, in fact, sleep intensified. An almost irresistible desire to sleep is one of the first symptoms to be observed. If the dose of poison imparted by the snake has been small, the desire may pass off or the sleep may not assume the form of coma, but in all serious cases it quickly assumes that form. *Vice versa* the deepest coma becomes sleep again, when the suspended function of the cortical centres is roused by strychnine injections. The insensible and completely paralysed patient usually announces the gradual return of consciousness by a few groans and uneasy movements and not unfrequently begins to snore, as in ordinary sleep, when a smart shake at the shoulder will rouse him into full consciousness. At other times this transition from coma back to sleep does not take place and consciousness returns quite suddenly, the persons opening their eyes and looking around them, dazed and bewildered, but perfectly conscious at once. When coma is fully established and the largest and most powerful motor-centres have succumbed to the insidious poison, general paresis becomes general paralysis and all the motor-centres of the body are in a condition of more or less suspended functional activity. This and this only is the condition of the centres, the whole secret of snake-poison, that has puzzled the human mind for ages and yet appears so simple when discovered at last. It is beautifully and strikingly illustrated in the phenomena before us. We have coma and complete general paralysis, every motor-nerve cell, from the highest psycho-motor one downwards, is thrown into a state of torpor and has ceased to discharge the life force that regulates every process of life and the entire absence of which inevitably must be death. Only weak, lingering currents are sent forth yet and put off the inevitable finale for a time. But the strychnine is injected and mark the change. It courses quickly to every one of the sleepers, for whom it also has an affinity, but the direct opposite to that of the deadly venom that has overpowered them. It touches them as if with the wand of a magician and orders them to awake and do their work. There is no disobeying the mandate, for it is founded on one of nature's unchangeable laws. Almost immediately the cells begin their work again, the life streams flow afresh, coma and paralysis vanish and within a very short time the subject of this beautiful experiment is snatched from the brink of the grave and restored to life and health.

The phenomena of sleep and coma as the result of a poison acting as a depressant of motor nerve force afford food for some interesting speculations, which, however, as more concerning the psychologist, the writer can only glance at here. It is evident that in the highest of psycho-motor centres, the organs of thought and of consciousness, the paresis of the lower centres assumes the form of sleep, and paralysis that of coma. Sleep, as a partial, and coma, as a complete, obliteration of thought and consciousness must, therefore, be intimately connected with motor nerve function, sleep being a reduction, coma a suppression of the function, or a suspension of thought. Ideation, to use J. S. Mill's very appropriate term for the thought process, appears to be effected by motor nerve currents or, at all events, to be accompanied by them and suspended with their suspension. The thinking principle, the nous within us, is no doubt more than mere nerve action, but it can, apparently, not manifest its presence without motor nerve cells in healthy action. Every thought, though not synonymous, is evidently synchronous with a current of motor nerve force, and it is not improbable that, by means of these currents, that silent transference of thought is effected from brain to brain, which modern psychology has demonstrated to be not only possible but actual under certain conditions. But further speculation on these interesting mysteries it would be out of place here to indulge in.

F. Action on Sensory Centres and the Reflexes

The sensory sphere remains comparatively unaffected in mild cases, and in the early stages of more serious ones, but when paresis has deepened into paralysis, sensation becomes ever more blunted, and with the advent of coma, of course, quite extinct. Reflexes, both superficial and deep ones, are also completely abolished at this period of the poisoning process, and the nerves of special sense do not react against any, even the strongest possible stimulation. The eye stares vacantly into a glaring light held close before it, and the widely dilated pupil shows no sign of reaction. The ear also appears deaf to any noise, and strong ammonia vapour is inhaled through the nose like the purest air, whilst pricking, beating, and even burning the skin elicit not a quiver of a muscle.

Feoktistow's experiments with regard to reflexes, more especially their restoration by strychnine, differ in their results entirely from Australian observations. Whilst we have no difficulty in restoring them with the drug on man as well as the domestic animals, his experiments on frogs were a failure, and merely showed a decided antagonism between the two poisons. He did not succeed in restoring the reflexes, and, instead of following up with experiments on the higher animals, he trusted implicitly to his results on frogs, and thus lost his opportunity.

G. Irregularities in the Action of Snake-poison

There is in the whole range of toxicology not a single condition known to us in which the symptoms, both in chronological order and in their strength and relation to each other, show as much variety as those of snake-poison. Experienced observers will agree with the writer that it is but rarely we find two cases of snakebite exactly alike in the symptoms they present. Some of these puzzling variations have already been alluded to, but it is necessary to consider them a little more in detail. Apart from quantitative differences in the poison imparted, they arise principally from the strange capriciousness with which the poison concentrates its action on special nerve centres and leaves others comparatively intact.

The nearest approach to regularity and orderly sequence of the symptoms, as described in the foregoing pages, we find in Australia after the bite of the tiger snake (*Hoplocephalus curtus*) and the brown snake (*Diemenia superciliosa*), more especially that of Queensland. Here we can trace the action of the poison distinctly from centre to centre, from the lowest part of the anterior cornua up to the cortex cerebri, and even throughout the sympathetic ganglia as far as they are patent to observation. The poison of these snakes is extremely diffusible and quickly absorbed. It spreads with rapidity and nearly equal force over all the motor centres, the symptoms following each other so quickly as almost to appear simultaneous, though, in reality, successive. But even the poison of these snakes leaves the arms only slightly paretic, when paralysis in all the other voluntary muscles is well pronounced, and does not paralyse them until coma has set in. It also touches the respiratory centre but slightly. Sometimes coma is light and the patients can be roused for a little while, at other times it is deep and lasts till death. But even greater variations are observed occasionally. In one very extraordinary case of tiger snakebite, the patient, a child of 9 years, remained conscious to the last, and after vomiting blood freely died under symptoms of heart failure. In rare cases the symptoms resemble those of cobra poison.

If we turn from these to the black snake (*Pseudechis porphyriacus*) a different picture presents itself. Its poison does not produce so deep a coma and often none at all. The patients generally feel drowsy and fall asleep, but are easily roused and sometimes awake spontaneously. There is also not the same amount of muscular paralysis. They are frequently able to walk a few steps with assistance and can move in bed, the arms especially being almost free from paresis. But the insidious poison none the less does its work, though its effects are less patent. It concentrates its action on the vaso-motor centre. The victims from hour to hour become more anæmic in appearance through increasing engorgement of the abdominal veins. Anæmia of the nerve-centres hastens the collapse, and from the combined effects of this and heart failure death takes place suddenly and quickly as if in a fainting fit. Here then we have an approach to the effects of viper poison which is also shown in the greater amount of swelling and effusion around the bite and in the bitten limb.

This approach is still closer in the poison of the death adder (*Acantophis antarctica*). There is generally much extravasation of blood locally. Muscular paralysis is also less pronounced, but sudden collapse from vaso-motor paralysis not unfrequently takes place, when the patients fully conscious are still able to sit up. That leading feature of viper poison, diapedesis with hæmorrhage, does not occur with either.

If we turn from Australian to Indian snakes, the peculiar tendency of the poison to concentrate its action on special nerve-centres becomes still more marked. The predilection of the cobra poison for the respiratory centre has already been dwelt on. More remarkable and strange is the action of the Indian viper-poison on the minute ganglia in the vaso-motor nerve ends, which control the capillary circulation, and by their paralysis bring about extensive hæmorrhage through diapedesis.

It is quite impossible for us with our present scanty knowledge to account for these peculiarities and irregularities in the action of a poison, which we know now to accomplish its destruction of animal life by one uniform design and principle of action. That the protean forms under which the poison-symptoms present themselves are one and all the result of reduction and suspension of motor nerve currents may now be accepted as a well proven and fully established scientific fact. But why the effects of one and the same cause are so varying in their appearance, why the poison of different varieties of snakes, and even that of the same variety under different circumstances, make such a capricious selection among the various motor nerve-centres we can not explain and probably never will. Chemical analysis of the dead poison, no matter how minutely and elaborately it may be effected, will probably never throw much light on the "why" of this strange puzzle, for the subtle phenomena of life are apt to elude the grasp of the analyst. We have to do with a poison transferred from one living organism into another one and modified in its action by the condition of the giver and the constitution and peculiarities of the recipient quite as much probably as by slight variations in its chemical composition. Accepting the "why" of these phenomena like that of many other ones, simply as a fact not to be accounted for at present, we must be content to know "how" they are effected, and, what is of more immediate and paramount importance to know, that we now have an antidote that will deal successfully with them all, that the convulsions and hæmorrhages of the Indian viper-poison and the asphyxia of that of the cobra will yield as readily to strychnine, when properly and boldly applied, as the coma and general paralysis following the bite of the deadly tiger snake.

THE ANTIDOTE

The theory of the action of snake-poison as that of a specific nerve-poison, depressing and more or less suspending the function of the motor nerve-centres throughout the body, has in the foregoing pages received a double proof of its correctness.

In the first place, all the symptoms the snake-poison produces have been passed in review, and shown to be fully explainable by this theory. On this ground alone it may be claimed to have been fully established; for it is an axiom in science that a theory on any subject must be accepted as correct, if it accounts satisfactorily for all the phenomena observable in connection with that subject by showing them to result from the operation of one law. The second inductive proof of the correctness of the writer's theory has been rendered by the experiments of Feoktistow on animals.

Science, however, demands that a theory thus established inductively must also stand the test of practical application or deduction. It says in the present case:—"Granting your theory to be correct, it is but a theory, which, however valuable it may be as a contribution to science, is of little value to mankind if you cannot apply it practically. If snake-poison merely acts as a depressant on motor nerve-cells without interfering with their structure, you must be able to counteract it by administering some drug or substance which acts as a powerful stimulant on these cells, if such a substance can be found."

It is another illustration of that wise adaptation of means to ends which, throughout the domain of nature, denotes the presence and rule of a Supreme Intelligence, that this substance has been provided for us by nature, though we have been long in finding it. Its discovery in strychnine, and its successful application as the long and vainly sought antidote to snake-poison, are glorious triumphs of scientific deduction.

Strychnine is the exact antithesis to snake-poison in its action. Under its influence every motor nerve-cell throughout the system sends forth stronger currents of nerve force than it does in its normal state. These currents run alike from cell to cell, and from cell to peripheral fibre, and act by means of the latter on all contractile, and especially all muscular tissue, causing contractions, which, after poisonous doses of the drug, assume the form of tetanic convulsions, provoked by the slightest touch or even noise in consequence of highly intensified reflex action.

Whilst, then, snake-poison, as we have seen, turns off the motor-batteries and reduces the volume and force of motor-nerve currents, strychnine, when following it as an antidote, turns them on again, acting with the unerring certainty of a chemical test, *if administered in sufficient quantity*. Purely physiological in its action, it neutralises the effects of the snake-poison, and announces, by unmistakable symptoms, when it has accomplished this task, and would, if continued, become a poison itself. Previous to this announcement its poisonous action is completely neutralised by the snake-poison, and the latter would therefore be equally as efficacious in strychnine-poisoning as strychnine is in snake-poisoning. Strychnine, in short, is the antidote *par excellence* of snake-poison, and cannot be surpassed by any other substance known to us.

With the symptoms following the introduction of the subtle ophidian virus into the human and animal system so markedly pointing to strychnine as the antidote, it appears a matter of surprise that it was not used as such before and that it was left to the writer to discover the antagonism between the two poisons. Misleading experiments with the drug on animals erroneously considered to be final in their results, together with confused and contradictory notions about the action of snake-poison, were the chief factors, already pointed out, that caused research on this important subject to remain for centuries so barren of results, and made even able investigators with more correct views than the rest, postpone the discovery of a physiological antidote to a more advanced state of science, when all the time it was lying ready at their hands.

It is self-evident from preceding statements, that in the treatment of snakebite with strychnine the ordinary doses must be greatly exceeded, and that its administration must be continued, even if the total quantity injected within an hour or two amounts to what in the absence of snake-poison would be a dangerous if not a fatal dose. Timidity in handling the drug is fraught with far more danger than a bold and fearless use of it. The few failures among its numerous successes recorded during the last four years in Australia were nearly all traceable to the antidote not having been injected in sufficient quantity. Even slight tetanic convulsions, which were noticed in a few cases, invariably passed off quickly. It should be borne in mind that of the two poisons warring with each other that of the snake is by far the most insidious and dangerous one, more especially in its effects on the vaso-motor centres. The latter are wrought very insidiously, and where they predominate require the most energetic use of the antidote, for whilst the timid practitioner after injecting as much strychnine as he deems safe stands idly by waiting for its effects, the snake virus, not checked by a sufficient quantity of it, continues its baneful work, drawing the blood mass into the paralysed abdominal veins and finally by arrested heart action bringing on sudden collapse. In such cases even some tetanic convulsions are of little danger and may actually be necessary to overcome the paralysis of the splanchnicus and with it that of the other vaso-motor centres.

Whilst then it must be laid down as a principle that the antidote should be administered freely and without regard to the quantity that may be required to develop symptoms of its own physiological action, the doses in which it is injected and the intervals between them must be left to the practitioner's judgment, as they depend in every case on the quantity of snake-poison absorbed, the time elapsed since its inception and the corresponding greater or lesser urgency of the symptoms. If the latter denote a large dose to have been imparted and it has been in the system for hours, delay is dangerous and nothing less than 16 minims of liq. strychnine P.B., in very urgent cases even 20 to 25 minims should be injected to any person over 15 years of age. Even children may require these large doses, as they are determined by the quantity of the poison they have to counteract and are kept in check by it. The action of the antidote is so prompt and decisive that not more than 15 to 20 minutes need to elapse, after the first injection, before further measures can be decided on. If the poisoning symptoms show no abatement by that time, a second injection of the same strength should be made promptly, and unless after it a decided improvement is perceptible, a third one after the same interval. As the action of strychnine when applied as antidote is not cumulative, no fear needs to be entertained of violent effects suddenly breaking out after these large doses repeated at short intervals. They are, so to say, swallowed up by the snake-poison and remain latent except in counteracting the latter. This has now been proven abundantly by scores of qualified observers in all parts of Australia, and still more by Banerjee in India. No hesitation, therefore, should be felt by medical men in other snake-infested countries to adopt the Australian treatment. It is seldom that more than half a grain of strychnine administered in 16m. doses of liq. strychniæ is required here to effectually counteract the venom and place its intended victim out of danger. Ligature and excision of the bitten skin have usually been practised and much of the poison eliminated before the antidote is applied. Our snakes, however, as already pointed out, with their shorter and merely grooved fangs, do not perforate the cellular tissue to such depth nor instil as large a quantity of poison as the cobras, kraits and vipers of India or the rattlesnake of America, all having perforated and much longer fangs and much more productive poison glands. Even if after the bite of a vigorous cobra, for instance, a ligature has been applied and the bitten part deeply excised, a comparatively large quantity of poison will probably be absorbed requiring much larger quantities of the antidote, perhaps grains of it, to effect a cure.

If under the influence of these large doses the symptoms abate, or if the latter are comparatively mild from the first, smaller doses of strychnine should be injected, say from 1/15th to 1/10th of a grain, but under all circumstances the rule that, distinct strychnia symptoms must be produced before the injections are discontinued, should never be departed from. This rule is a perfectly safe one, for its observance entails no danger, a few muscular spasms or even slight tetanic convulsions being easily subdued and harmless as compared with that most insidious condition exemplified in case No. 1, cited below, the first one treated with strychnine by the writer, who, having no experience in the treatment, did not administer quite enough strychnine. The patient, after apparently recovering from a moribund condition and being able to walk and even to mount a horse, remained partly under the influence of the poison and succumbed to it during sleep, when, according to subsequent experience, one more injection would have saved him.

The tendency to relapses is always great when much snake-poison has been absorbed. Apparently yielding to the antidote for a time, the insidious venom, after a shorter or longer interval, during which it appears to have been conquered, all at once re-asserts its presence, and has to be met by such fresh injections, regardless of the quantity of strychnine previously administered, but the amount required in most relapses is not a large one. The writer formerly inclined to the belief that the strain thus put on the delicate nerve-cells would limit the usefulness of the antidote to cases requiring not much above a grain. Knowing the Indian snakes to impart to their victims such comparatively large quantities of venom, he had strong misgivings as to his method standing the severe test of Indian practice; and it was most fortunate for this method that its first practical application in India was made by a gentleman who, whilst thoroughly familiar with its principles and convinced of their correctness, had the courage to apply them fearlessly by injecting what to us Australians appear enormous quantities, ranging as they do up to three and four grains per patient. Dr. Banerjee's eight cases, all successful, and of which the most important one, relating to the much and justly dreaded Duboia Russellii, was published in the November number of the *Australasian Medical Gazette*, settled the treatment of snakebite in India as well as elsewhere. If the poison of Bungarus coeruleus, Echis carinata, and Duboia Russellii can be successfully counteracted, and if for this purpose four grains of strychnine can be injected with perfect impunity, it may be inferred with certainty that the poison of the cobra, fer-de-lance, and the rattlesnake—in fact, of any snake known to us will be found amenable to the antidote, and that, if four grains can be injected with safety, we may venture on six and eight grains, if they are required. In those cases only where the long fangs of these snakes perforate into a vein, and a large quantity of the venom injected into the blood-stream overpowers the nerve-centres so as to make death imminent, if not almost instantaneous, the subcutaneous injections may be found of little use. Here intravenous injections of half a grain and even one grain doses would appear to be indicated, and might yet fan the flame of life afresh, even when respiration and pulse at wrist have already ceased. We have seen both these functions extinct in Australia and restored by comparatively small doses of the antidote, and can see no reason why a more energetic use of it should not restore them in India.

Considering the terrible mortality from snakebite in India, Dr. Banerjee's merit in being the first to introduce the strychnine treatment there is of a very high order, and his grateful countrymen will ever cherish his memory. When his Excellency the Viceroy had been appealed to in vain by the writer, and the adoption of his method in India urged through two Australian Governors, a native of India has stepped forward and taken the first step towards alleviating an evil that has hurried over two millions of his countrymen in every century to an untimely grave.

The cases as reported by him to the *Australasian Medical Gazette* are cited below.

CASES

If the deductions and conclusions set forth in the foregoing chapters are correct, it may be justly contended that all cases of snakebite treated with strychnine should invariably end in recovery if the antidote is properly applied, according to the rules above detailed. This contention the writer fully and cordially endorses. Given the largest amount of poison a snake can give off at one bite, strychnine injected in time and sufficient quantity—either by the hypodermic, or, if urgent, by the intravenous method—must rouse the dormant nerve-cells into action, as long as the vital functions are not completely extinct. Wherever it fails, the fault lies with the operator not injecting it in sufficient quantity—a fault committed by the writer himself in his first case.

The following condensed accounts of fifty cases treated in Australia, and eight in India, the writer has taken mostly from the *Australasian Medical Gazette*. Two of these only are from his own practice; others were kindly communicated to him by his colleagues. It is not claimed that all these cases were rescues from certain death. Some of them undoubtedly were, others would have recovered under some other treatment or no treatment at all; but in none of them would recovery have been so rapid and complete. The two poisons are thrown out together, and no ill-effects of either are experienced beyond a certain degree of weakness, which passes off quickly. This is a boon to be appreciated fully by those only who have gone through the slow, lingering, and painful process of convalescence from snakebite as formerly treated, with its deadly languor and weariness, making life itself a burden and all physical and mental exertion impossible.

> Case 1.—A. H., 15 years old, a farm labourer, was bitten
> on the right index finger whilst feeling for a rabbit in a
> burrow. Did not see the snake nor suspect snakebite, but
> collapsed helplessly in a few minutes after returning to his
> work. The writer saw him three hours after the accident. He
> was then completely paralysed and in deep coma; pupils
> widely dilated and not reacting to light; sense of sight and
> hearing dead; heart action extremely feeble; pulse small,

thread-like, and scarcely countable; respiration quick and shallow; skin blanched and very cold. Seeing him dragged along the road between two men, had him quickly carried to the next house, and injected 20 minims of liq. strychnine. Only a groan or two and a slight improvement in the pulse, indicating a change in his condition, gave him a second injection about twenty minutes after the first one. A change for the better then became rapidly conspicuous. The pulse gained in strength from minute to minute, respiration became deeper, and the coma was visibly reduced to mere sleep, from which there was no difficulty in rousing him to full consciousness by a vigorous shake of the shoulders. This marvellous change was brought about within forty minutes; and this being the first case to which the writer had applied his theory by injecting strychnine, its unparalleled success exceeded his most sanguine expectations, but unfortunately also lulled him into a false sense of security, which proved disastrous to his patient. Not knowing then as he does now that the snake-poison after having been subdued by the antidote is not thrown out of the system as quickly as the strychnine, and is therefore apt to re-assert itself, he allowed another urgent engagement to take him away from the lad after watching him for two hours and actually taking the evening tea with him. His instructions to the mother not to let her son go to sleep and to watch him carefully for the slightest sign of the return of symptoms, were unfortunately disobeyed. Both mother and son went to sleep, deeming all danger over. During this sleep the lad again relapsed into coma and was found so at daylight. All attempts to rouse him were fruitless, and he died before the messenger intended for me had time to saddle a horse. The death of the unfortunate lad, however, has saved some lives since. It taught the writer the lesson never to trust to the apparent success of the antidote until it shows distinct signs of its own physiological action, and even then to watch his patients carefully for the first twenty-four hours, and let them sleep for short periods only.

Case 2.—A.H., a vigorous girl of 20 years, bitten above the left ankle by a snake in some long grass, and therefore not identified. Had applied two tight ligatures above the bite, ran home and got her mother to cut out the bitten skin, showing two distinct punctures. Seen within an hour after the bite the girl presented distinct, but moderate symptoms, deadly paleness, very cold skin, small frequent pulse, and a peculiar feeling of agony about the heart, just able to sit upright, but unable to walk. All symptoms increased rapidly after writer cut ligatures. She reeled from side to side, and suddenly fell forward as if in a swoon. Injected 1/6th grain of strychnine and, as she did not lose consciousness, was able to watch the interesting and rapid effect of the antidote. It had not been injected more than five minutes when slight colour returned to the cheeks, naturally very red. Patient then stated that the distressing feeling about the heart was getting less and also that of drowsiness. From minute to minute her condition improved, and in about ten she was able to rise and walk a few steps. Profiting, however, by the lesson his first case had given him, the writer did not trust to her apparent recovery, but seeing that much of the poison had been eliminated by the prompt measures taken before he saw her, he injected only 1/12th of a grain, which produced slight muscular spasms. Careful precautions were taken in this case against a relapse, but none took place, and when visited next morning the girl declared herself as well as ever she had been in her life.

The following notes of two cases of tiger snake bite (*Hoplocephalus curtus*), treated with strychnine, were read by Dr. Thwaites before the Intercolonial Medical Congress of 1889. This gentleman, a young practitioner just entering practice, had the courage to use the antidote according to the writer's directions in spite of the hostile criticisms of his seniors in the profession and even his own university teachers, and thereby not only saved two valuable lives, but also set a praiseworthy example, which was soon followed by others. The writer gives the notes abbreviated.

Case 3.—J. B., a strong, robust labourer, bitten by a tiger snake on the back of right hand. Killed the snake, which hung on to the hand and was with some difficulty shaken off. Made slight incision through the punctures and tied a rag round the wrist, but too loosely to check circulation; then started for the next neighbour's house, distant a mile, which he reached with difficulty, staggering like a drunken man when he arrived. The bitten skin was here excised, whisky administered and patient sent on in a buggy, but distance being 30 miles to Dr. Thwaites' residence, a messenger on horseback galloped ahead to get Dr. Thwaites to meet buggy on road. The latter writes: "I met buggy four miles from my residence. Patient had to be held up on the seat of the vehicle between two men. He had not spoken for some time, pulse very weak, pupils greatly dilated, face very pale. I injected 10 minims of liq. strychnine P.B. at once, and in a few minutes noticed some improvement. He now answered when spoken to, his pulse became stronger, and he could walk a few steps. This was at 5.30 p.m., and he kept up fairly well till 8.15, when he collapsed completely. I now injected 20 minims of liq. strychniæ, which in a short time brought him round; but at 9.15 another relapse took place, when a third injection of 15 m. was made. This was followed by slight twitching about the face and neck, after which improvement and recovery were uninterrupted."

Dr. Thwaites' second case is even more remarkable and telling. When the girl, after a journey of 30 miles, was carried into his surgery, she appeared to be dead, and a second medical man, who happened to be present, declared her to be so, and all attempts to revive her useless.

Case 4.—A. D., aged 15 years, a schoolgirl, bitten by a vigorous tiger-snake on the outside of left leg, the snake also holding on for some time. She at once tightened her garter above the knee and ran home, a distance of three-quarters of a mile. The bitten skin was at once excised, another firm ligature applied, whisky administered, and a hurried start made for Dr. Thwaites', distant 30 miles,

where she arrived five hours after accident. The latter
writes:—"She was then pulseless at wrists, cold as a stone,
and with pupils insensible to light. I could not perceive
any respiration, but felt the heart yet faintly fluttering. She
was to all appearances just on the point of death. I injected
at once 17 minims of liq. strychniæ. In about two minutes
she sighed, and then began to breathe in a jerky manner. In
about ten minutes, on my pulling her hair, she opened her
eyes and looked around, but could not recognise any one.
Pupils now acted to stimulus of light. In a short time she
could speak when spoken to, but not see at any distance.
Her sight gradually returned completely; she kept on
improving, and in four to five hours after the one injection
she seemed quite well, but rather weak. I gave small doses
of stimulants till morning, and did not let her go to sleep
till next evening. She suffered no relapse, and her recovery
was complete."

Case 5.—This remarkable case was not published in the
medical press, but in many of the papers of Queensland,
where it created much sensation. The writer is indebted
for an account of it to Dr. Thwaites, who vouches for its
correctness. It appears that this gentleman acquainted
the well-known explorer of Northern Queensland, Mr.
Johnstone, who is his uncle, and now police magistrate at
Maryborough, Queensland, with his success in treating
snakebite with strychnine. Mr. Johnstone, who during his
explorations had seen much of snakebite and many deaths
from it, wrote rather incredulously in reply, stating that
our southern snakes were innocuous in comparison with
those of the north; and that, having seen twelve persons
bitten and die by the deadly brown snake of the north
(*Diemenia superciliosa*), he must withhold his belief in
the new antidote until he had witnessed a case of brown
snakebite cured by it or reported on good authority. This
desire he had quickly gratified, and by a strange fatality
in his own person. Whilst taking his children for a walk
in the bush a few weeks afterwards he stepped aside the
path to pluck a flower from a bush, and in doing so was

bitten on the leg by a vigorous brown snake. He at once
applied a ligature, and had the punctures sucked by an
aboriginal, but became comatose before he reached home.
Three medical men were summoned in haste, injected
ammonia into several veins, and finally had to resort to
artificial respiration, declaring the case a hopeless one. In
this extremity Mrs Johnstone rushed to a fourth one, who
had seen Dr. Thwaites' letter, and discussed its contents
with her husband in her presence. This gentleman—Dr.
Garde—laid up in bed, quickly furnished the lady with liq.
strychniæ, accompanied by the request to his colleagues
to inject it freely. She came back to her husband's bedside,
when artificial respiration was about to be given up, but the
very first injection rendered it no longer necessary and two
more restored Mr. Johnstone completely. Saving the life of
this highly respected and popular functionary, who was
the first in Queensland treated with the antidote, paved
the way for it in that colony, where it is most needed and is
now highly appreciated.

These five cases, thoroughly typical of the effects of
strychnine in snakebite, are almost in themselves sufficient
to bear out the correctness of the writer's deductions, but
for the benefit of a certain class of rigorously incredulous
scientists, who would not be satisfied with five cases,
the writer submits 45 more and in addition to these—
last but not least—Dr. Bannerjee's eight Indian cases.
They are all well authenticated, being mostly taken from
the *Australasian Medical Gazette* or from private notes, but
to avoid useless repetition the greater part of them will be
merely cited and only the more remarkable ones be given
in detail. Whether in the face of this formidable array of
evidence that blind incredulity and senseless opposition,
usually blocking the way of every new discovery, will
at last give way, remains to be seen. The writer has had
his full share of them, and but for the valuable aid he
received from the Hon. Dr. Creed, the able editor of the *A.
M. Gazette*, would probably be struggling yet for the
introduction of his antidote. When it is considered that,

in spite of such evidence as here produced, his discovery
has as yet received no official recognition from any of
the Australian medical authorities, and that even now
there are medical men who can write such effusions as
that of Dr. T. L. Bancroft, of Brisbane, beginning with
the words: "It is deplorable to still see recorded cases of
snakebite treated with strychnine, &c.," (see *Gazette* for
July, 1892)—the attitude assumed from the first by Dr.
Creed and his unfailing advocacy of the antidote can not
be too highly appreciated and lay both the writer and the
public under a debt of deep gratitude to him. But for his
early recognition of the soundness of the writer's theory
and treatment of snakebite many valuable lives now
saved would have been lost. As early as June, 1889, Dr.
Creed wrote in an editorial: "We desire to call the special
attention of the profession to Dr. Mueller's papers on the
pathology and cure of snakebite, published in our issues
for Nov., Dec., Feb, April and May last, and to press
upon them the justice and, we submit, the necessity of
extremely careful consideration of his theory and of the
results shown in the cases in which, acting on it, he has
used hypodermic injections of strychnine for the treatment
of snakebite. We formerly expressed our concurrence in
the opinion of Sir Joseph Fayrer, who wrote: 'I do not say
that a physiological antidote is impossible, all I assert is,
that it is not yet found.' We are indeed pleased to state
that we believe such an antidote is now found and that
Dr. Mueller is the happy discoverer. We are of opinion
that his theory as to the pathological changes set up in the
human system by the injection of snake-poison is a sound
one and that the treatment he has suggested and used is
correct and proper, and the one likely to avert death in
cases of snakebite, which would otherwise in all probability
prove fatal. We therefore press the use of hypodermic
injections of strychnia in the manner described by him
upon the attention of practitioners who may have to treat
cases in which the symptoms present are the result of
snake or dangerous insect poison, and think that, should
the patients die without its having been used, all will not

have been done to save life that might have been." Without such utterances repeated from time to time and without the ample space always allowed in the *Gazette* to the subject, a record like that now submitted would not have been possible.

Case 6.—P. Evans, a girl of 20 years, bitten on wrist by a brown snake. Symptoms—Staggering gait, drowsiness, &c. Only 1/16th grain in four injections. Notes furnished by Drs. Mahoney and Kennedy, of Albury.

Case 7.—W. Thiplin, a labourer, bitten on hand by brown snake. Three injections. Notes by Dr. Baird of Healesville.

Case 8.—Luke Dewhurst, labourer, bitten on hand by tiger snake. Cured by one injection of m. xv. liq. strychniæ after ammonia had failed. Notes by Dr. Dutton, of Lillydale.

Case 9.—P. Moroney, labourer, bitten on thigh at night, snake not identified. Cured by three injections of 1/12th grain each. Notes by Dr. Pardey, of Myrtleford.

Case 10.—Mrs. Skinner, bitten on thigh, at Carrum. Treated by Dr. Verity.

Case 11.—Child of Mr. Weeks, aged three years. Treated by Dr. Degner, of Myrtleford.

Case 12.—Annie Rankin, servant, at Corowa. Treated by local chemist.

Case 13.—Child of Mr. F. Daniels, of Mount Kent, Queensland, *only two years old*, bitten by a death adder on fourth finger of left hand, the snake found clinging to finger. Ligature applied and finger chopped off, but condition of child very precarious when admitted to Toowoomba Hospital, after a night's journey, at daylight, in complete collapse. Pronounced out of danger by Dr. Hunt, the house-surgeon, at 10.30 and taken home in the afternoon. Notes not furnished.

Case 14.—Reported by Dr. Pain, of Allora, Queensland. Symptoms serious. Four injections of m. xv., x., viii. and vii.

Case 15.—Reported by Dr. Garde, of Maryborough, Queensland, girl of 13 years, bitten by brown snake, requiring only two injections of m. xv. and x.

Case 16.—Reported by Dr. St. George Queely, of Maytown, Queensland, lad of 19 years, bitten by black snake, symptoms serious. Four injections of m. xv., xv., xx., and xv., total 65 minims of liq. strych. P.B. injected within less than two hours, muscular spasms appearing after last injection. Patient made rapid recovery, riding home, a distance of 16 miles, within a few hours after treatment.

Case 17.—Reported by Dr. Ray, of Seymour, severe bite of a tiger snake. Within six hours 4/5th of a grain administered subcutaneously, besides a considerable quantity given by the mouth. Patient made a good recovery. "Every injection after the second one," Dr. Ray reports, "having a distinct effect within three or four minutes, and lasting from one to one and a half hours before tendency to coma returned."

Case 18.—Very remarkable. Read by Dr. Forbes, medical officer of hospital, Charters Towers, Queensland, before the North Queensland Medical Society. Boy, 6 years old, was admitted to hospital at 9 p.m. on 27th October, 1890, bitten on foot by a death adder, which was killed and identified. Dr. Forbes reports: When seen by me, two hours after the accident, he was sitting on his mother's knee with his head hanging on one side, but quite conscious, and answering questions rationally, pupils widely dilated with almost no reaction to light, pulse very fast and soft, &c. Thinking his condition might be due to fear I hesitated to use strychnine. So, ordering strong coffee, I hurried to attend an accident case just admitted with severe hæmorrhage, and left the boy in charge of a nurse, with orders to call me at once if she saw any change. I had scarcely been away 15 minutes when the father rushed in saying his boy was dead, and indeed his statement seemed but too true. The child was lying quite limp, face blue, eyes half shut, extremities very cold, no pulse perceptible, no respiration visible. I at once injected m. x. of liq. strychniæ P.B. and made artificial respiration. He soon began to improve, and in about 20 minutes was able to speak. He was watched all night, but suffered no relapse, and was discharged on the next day.

Cases 19 to 21, reported by Dr. Weekes, of Lithgow, N.S.W. Dr. Weekes writes:—"Within the last year I have had three cases under my care, all bitten by black snakes, and all in about the same place, on the outside of the calf of the leg. The patients were all comatose, exhibiting all the usual symptoms of snakebite-poisoning, and in one, my last case, *the patient had convulsions.* In all of them I made hypodermic injections of m. xv. liq. strych., and the effects were most marked, the patients being completely roused and becoming quite sensible and rational each time," &c.

Case 22.—Mrs. Ryan, of Oberon, N.S.W., bitten on leg by tiger snake, comatose and nearly pulseless after three hours, treated by Dr. Kingsburry, amount of strychnine not stated.

Case 23.—Benjamin Childs, bitten on finger by death adder, treated by Dr. Campbell, of Grafton, N.S.W.

Case 24.—Rather remarkable. Reported by Dr. Lloyd Parry, of Emmaville, N.S.W., in *Gazette* of March, 1891, and further particulars in private correspondence with writer. A Chinese miner, aged 30 years, was bitten on the back of the foot by a death adder. His mates, deeming medical aid useless, did not send for Dr. Parry until death was imminent, and then only with a view of getting a certificate of death, and avoiding autopsy and inquest. When seen, three hours after infliction of bite, the man was deeply comatose and pulseless, skin icy cold, pupils dilated and insensible to light, lower jaw hanging down and tongue protruding, respiration scarcely perceptible. He was in fact so near death that this event was expected to take place from minute to minute. In order to task the antidote to the utmost, Dr. Parry cut the tight ligature without excising the bitten skin and then injected xv. of liq. st. P.B. To his surprise in a few minutes the man began to groan and very soon afterwards became conscious. Dr. Parry then watched him carefully and in about an hour found coma returning, when another injection was made and roused him for good. There was much swelling and effusion in the leg, but no ill effects followed.

In this case, judging from the comparatively small quantity of the antidote required, only a small amount of poison had been imparted, the bite being on the back of the foot, where the fangs cannot penetrate deeply. Still there can be no doubt that even this small quantity of the justly dreaded death adder poison would have proved fatal, if it had not been counteracted by the antidote.

Case 25, reported from Tasmania by Dr. Holmes, of Launceston, presents different features, showing the very large quantity of the antidote sometimes required. After describing the condition of his patient, a Mrs. Frazer, of St. Leonards, Dr. Holmes writes:—"From her desperate condition I thought it too late for the ammonia treatment and decided on injecting liq. strychniæ. At 12.30 p.m. injected m. xv, at 1.40, m. xv., at 2.10, m. xv., at 2.40, m. xv., and 3.10, m. xv., at 4 p.m., m. x., and at 5, m. x. A few minutes after the last dose I noticed the physiological action of the drug and desisted from injecting. At 8 p.m. she seemed almost well, pupils normal in size and reacting well, was not sleepy and could swallow easily. The patient made a good recovery."

This is the largest quantity of strychnine that has been required in Australia, namely, 126 minims of liq. strych., or 1-1/9th gr. injected in less than five hours, with the most beneficial result. Surely the most cynical scepticism must give in to such facts.

Case 26.—Reported by Dr. MacDonald, of Murwillumbah, N.S.W. Mr. S., bitten on leg by a black snake. Coma, complete paralysis, chin hanging down to sternum, pupils dilated, &c. An injection of m. xv. had no effect; one of m. xx. very little. After a third one of m. x. patient suddenly became conscious, could walk without assistance, and in half an hour was sent to bed perfectly recovered.

Case 27.—Reported by Dr. Yeatman, of Auburn, South Australia. Mr. D., a farmer, aged 45 years, bitten on thumb; snake not named; cured by three injections of only m. v. each. Convulsions lasting for an hour came on three hours after treatment—a very rare occurrence—by Dr. Yeatman erroneously ascribed to the strychnine, which in so small a dose would not have produced them in the absence of snake-poison.

Case 28.—Reported by officer in charge of police at Grenfell. Boy of 6 years, bitten by brown snake, and treated by Dr. Rygate.

Case 29.—W. Toomer, aged 19, bitten by tiger snake on thumb and index finger, and not treated until 9-1/2 hours after bite, having a long distance to travel. Recovery very slow through timid use of antidote, five injections of 1/30th grain having but little effect, until one of 1/10th restored him. Treated by Dr. Stokes, of Echuca.

Case 30.—Reported by Dr. Bennett, surgeon, Gulgong Hospital, N.S.W. Mrs. Mears admitted to hospital comatose and pulseless, nothing having been done to check absorption. The intravenous injection of ammonia failing to rouse her, m. xv. of liq. strych. were injected, when pulse returned, but coma continued. After a second injection of m. xv. she suddenly became quite conscious, and in an hour was fully restored.

Case 31.—Reported by Dr. Mead, of Quirindi, N.S.W. John Simson, aged 15 years, bitten by a death adder on forefinger of right hand. Dr. Mead living 50 miles away, and the lad collapsing, a layman, Mr. Robert Simson, had to undertake treatment, and injected during the night m. 150 of a one in 240 solution of strychnine, equal to 5/8ths of a grain. Dr. Mead, finding the lad conscious and only a little drowsy, did not inject any more strychnine until 2 p.m., when a relapse took place. He then injected m. viii. of liq. str. P. B., and in half an hour m. vii. more. The last injection produced slight muscular twitchings, and subdued the snake-poison effectually, the lad making a good recovery.

The total quantity used in 13 injections was over three-quarters of a grain within 18 hours.

Case 32.—This case is another instance of the successful use of the antidote by a layman, and can be verified by the writer, who saw the patient, a girl of 14 years, after her father had carried out the treatment successfully. The girl had been bitten by a large brown snake whilst walking through a paddock, and very soon afterwards lost the use of her legs, and for a time also her eyesight. The symptoms being so very alarming, and the girl at a distance of 35 miles from the writer's residence, the father at once injected 1/12th of a grain of strychnine, and in a very short time another 1/12th. The child then rallied somewhat, and a start was made to bring her in, the father taking the precaution of bringing the antidote-case with him. This was fortunate, for the child collapsed several times, and each time had to be roused by an injection before reaching the writer. When finally she presented herself, walking into the writer's surgery with a firm step, not a trace could be discovered either of the strychnine, of which nearly half a grain had been injected, nor of the snake-poison, also imparted no doubt in a fatal dose. The two punctures on her leg, testifying to the size of the snake that had bitten her, were the only tokens of the ordeal she had gone through; and the only task remaining for the writer was to congratulate her father (Mr. James Trebilcock, a farmer, of Tawanga), on the plucky manner in which he had carried out the treatment, and see to the child being properly watched during the night in case of a relapse taking place. None, however, occurred, and she left next morning perfectly well. Cases of this kind, in which no doctor is called in, are frequently reported to the writer, who finds that laymen are even more successful because less timid than many medical men.

Case 33.—Joseph Cartledge, bitten on calf of leg by a black snake, was treated by Dr. Browne, of Sale, five hours after accident. Two injections of 1/8th grain each used.

Case 34.—Miss Davie, teacher, at Nerung, Queensland, treated by Dr. Hannah, of Southport. Particulars not given.

Case 35.—Mrs. Rogers, of Bulu Bulu, Gippsland, bitten on finger by tiger snake, and treated by Dr. Trampy, first with intravenous injections of ammonia, which had no effect, and when sinking with strychnine injections, which had almost immediate effect, and in a few hours placed her out of danger.

Case 36.—Son of Mr. J. Beveridge, squatter, of Glengower, treated successfully by Dr. Andrew, of Clunes, with strychnine injections.

Case 37.—Theresa Byrne, aged 14 years, bitten whilst bathing, snake not seen. Treated by Dr. Cuppaidge, of Normanby, Queensland. Only 18 minims of L. S. required.

Case 38.—Mr. Bullock, of Tenterfield, N.S.W., bitten by black snake and treated by Dr. Morice.

Case 39.—A boy, J. Taylor, bitten at Mount Keat, agricultural settlement, Queensland, by a black snake, and treated successfully by a layman, Mr. James Daniels.

Case 40.—George Neilson, a Danish miner, bitten by a tiger snake whilst bathing. Case reported by Dr. Gamble, of Walhalla. Forty minims of liq. strych. required; recovery complete next morning.

Cases 41 and 42, reported by Dr. Helsham, of Richmond, N.S.W. In one of these where, judging from the symptoms, a large dose of snake-poison had been absorbed, but very small doses of strychnine were injected, convulsions set in, *whilst coma was still present*, and lasted for two hours. Though semi-tetanic in appearance they were erroneously ascribed to m. xxvi. of liq. strychniæ, which at the time of their appearance had not removed the symptoms of snake-poison. They were evidently produced by the latter and quite on a par with those occasionally occurring in man before the strychnine is administered, and almost invariably in dogs. As long as coma is present with other

symptoms denoting the snake-poison to be in active
operation, such convulsions rather call for the antidote,
than contra indicate its use, for the strychnine never
produces them until it has completely conquered the snake-
poison, and even then they are always preceded by local
spasms and never set in suddenly. Timid medical men,
when administering the antidote and anxiously watching
for the dreaded strychnine effects, are too apt to see them in
the slightest irregular muscular action.

Case 43, reported by Dr. Johnson, of Avoca, patient bitten
by a tiger snake, was comatose, pulseless, with very
shallow respiration, &c., and restored by three injections of
m. xvi., xv. and x. within less than three hours.

Case 44.—Reported in *Australian Journal of Pharmacy*,
from Tasmania, treated by Dr. Tofft, of Campbell Town.
The report concludes: We have had some fatal cases of
snakebite already this season, and the successful treatment
in the above case has created a strong feeling in favour of
strychnine in such emergencies.

Cases 45 to 49.—Reported by Dr. Alex. Barber to *A.M.
Gazette*. He writes: "During the last year I treated four cases
of snakebite successfully with strychnine. In one of these, a
bite of a brown snake, I injected three doses of m. xx. each
of liq. strych. P.B., in all over half a grain, in one hour."

Case 50.—Reported by Dr. Barrington, of Benalla (Vic.), bite
of tiger snake, symptoms moderate. Completely removed
in three hours by 57 minims of liq. strych. P.B.

*Notes of eight cases as reported to the "Australasian Medical
Gazette" for July and November, 1892, by R. P. Banerjee, B.A.,
G.B.M.S.L., Medical Officer, Salt Mines, Pachhadra, Rajputana,
India:—*

Case 1.—Bhagwan Singh, aged 30, Hindu male, Sepoy,
E. T. Force, was bitten by a viperine snake (*echis carinata*)
at 4 p.m. 10th June, 1892, in the dorsum of left foot. He
was removed to the hospital, tight ligature applied, and
with the following symptoms:—Heaviness of both legs,

staggered if allowed to walk, giddiness, sense of sinking at the pit of the stomach, bleeding from mucous surfaces and old scars; soon fell swooning.

Treatment.—The punctures incised, and blood let out, one-twelfth of a grain of strychniæ; acetas hypodermically injected. Again, the insensibility not gone after 30 minutes, another dose given, and so repeated the third time. The *bleeding stopped* and the man recovered his senses, but could not raise himself to talk. Many more doses were given under the skin, with hour intervals, and the man recovered the next day; but he was much exhausted and treated for weakness three days, and discharged to duty on the 14th. Punctures were distinct, symptoms well developed. Took *one and a half grains* of strychnine to effect cure, leaving no after effects of the drug or poison.

Case 2.—Sadig Husain, a Mussulman boy, aged 12 years, bitten on the right ankle, just below the inner malleolus, by *echis carinata* (Khapar) on the 5th August, 1891, brought in with usual symptoms, as before.

Treatment as before. This case took only one-fourth grain of strych. acet. The boy was weak and sickly. He was discharged cured on the third day, *i.e.*, 17th August, 1891.

Case 3.—Nathey Khan, Mussulman, customs peon, aged 35 years, robust and strong, bitten by *echis carinata* (yellow variety). Punctures were on the left ankle, over the outer malleolus. Symptoms as before given.

Treatment as before stated. This case took as much as one and three quarter grains of strych. acet. Was admitted on the 9th August, 1891, and discharged on the 12th August, 1891, cured and fit for duty.

Case 4.—Musamat Jewai, Hindu female, a labourer, age 40, strong built. Bitten by kerait (*Bungarus coeruleus*), about 2-1/2 feet long, above the left knee joint; ligature below the hip was used, but all the symptoms were present and the patient was insensible. Cyanotic marks were seen on the arms, abdomen, back and neck. At first all hopes of recovery were given up, but attempts were made to see if anything could do good.

Treatment.—Punctures scarified and cupping applied. Repeated doses of strychnine acetas hypodermically given, but in *quarter grain* doses. It seemed marvellous. The cyanotic patches in the skin gradually faded away and the body became warmer. It was wondered if the person had expired, but suddenly the woman called for a drink of cold water to bathe her dry and parching mouth. This was done and she recovered sense. She was admitted on the 3rd September, 1891, and discharged on the 10th. Took *three grains* of acetate of strychnine to effect a cure.

Case 5.—Paroati Devi, Hindu female, aged 67 years, healthy constitution. Bitten on big toe of left foot on 10th September, 1891, symptoms were as preceding. The wound was cauterised.

Treatment.—Strychnia was given very cautiously, as the patient was over-aged, the degeneration of the heart kept in view—1/10 grain eventually showed the peculiar strychnine symptoms. The patient was cured in two days and discharged cured on the third day, 14th September, 1891. This patient took in all *one and a half grains* of acetate of strychnia.

Case 6.—Maya Swuper, aged 38 years, bitten by echis carinata (without dots) on the lower third of the left leg, on the outside of it. Mucous membrane of the mouth, eyes, nostrils, ears, and urinary passages all bled profusely. Urine had clots in it and symptoms resembled those in the first case.

Treated with strychnine and recovered in four days. Was admitted on the 14th September, 1891, and discharged to duty on the 18th September, 1891. Took in all *three grains* to effect cure.

Case 7.—Avghunandan, customs semadar, aged 55 years, Hindu male. Bitten at 8 a.m. on the 29th March, 1892, by echis carinata (brown variety) on the right foot near the cuboid bone. The punctures were distinct and the symptoms like those of case 1. Bleeding was profuse in this case.

Treatment.—Strychnine acetas injected *in quarter grain* doses under the skin and repeated as often as desirable. Patient recovered after the sixth day and took in *all four grains of strych. acet.* in six days. Only the bitten leg had erysipelatous inflammation, which had to be treated afterwards, but the man was quite safe.

Remarks.—In connection with echis bites one peculiar symptom was always noticed, namely, the free oozing of blood from mucous surfaces and old scars of wounds. The power of co-ordination was very much affected from the first setting in of other symptoms. Usually after 24 hours symptoms showed a relapse. In the treatment with strychnia neither the symptoms of the drug nor of the snake-poison ever showed themselves afterwards. Both seemed to neutralise each other. Bungarus coeruleus, or kerait-bite, had its own peculiar symptoms of cyanotic patches and insensibility, swooning and stertorous breathing. The true comatose state was not present in any, but only a slight one noticed in cases 4 and 5. The other cases were generally delirious in the beginning.

Case 8.—Dr. Banerjee communicated this case to the *Australasian Medical Gazette* separately and quite recently, November, 1892. It is, of all his cases, the most important one. He writes:—"The following case increases my number to eight, and should clear away prejudice and prepossessed ideas, as strychnine saved this case, a bite of *Duboia Russellii*. This snake is admitted by all hands to be virulently poisonous, and the poison is said to be even more virulent than that of the dreaded cobra:"—

Rahimudden, aged 43, Mussulman, customs peon, admitted for treatment of snakebite on the 13th September, 1892, at 10.45 p.m., to the North India Salt Revenue Hospital, Pachhadra, Rajputana, India, and put under my treatment.

History of the Case.—The man is of strong build and healthy constitution. While on duty he went round the salt pit, near his beat. Suddenly he felt a prick on his foot, and, suspecting snakebite, struck out with a bamboo stick he carried in his hand, and heard the snake make a loud noise. He at once tore a piece of cloth from his turban, and tied it tightly above the right ankle joint round the leg, then tried to kill the snake, but could not do so with certainty, as it was dark. He reported the case to his superiors, and was carried to the hospital. Bitten at 9.30 p.m.; admitted at 10.45 p.m.

Present Symptoms.—Patient was delirious, and could not understand what was told him; body cold and covered with perspiration; breathing hurried, with a low rattle at the end of expiration; mouth, tongue, and palate all dry; tongue leather-like and cracked, and felt cold; tickling of throat, not exciting vomiting; pupils dilated; conjunctiva congested; pulse 95; patient talked, or rather muttered, with difficulty; could not tolerate strong light or loud noise; the mucous membrane of the mouth showed irregular dark patches of ecchymosed blood.

The right foot was swollen, and in a line between ankle and knuckle of big toe showed two punctures—one deep and bleeding, and surrounded by ecchymosis; the other one below this, more superficial, the blood oozing thin and not coagulating. Received, at 10.45 p.m., 1/12th grain of strychnine in left arm. At 11 p.m., the same dose; breathing the same, but no rattle; stupor rather deepening; incoherency increasing. At 11.15, the same dose; breathing easier; stupor the same; pulse, 85; temp, 97.6; delirious at times, and moaning with inarticulate cries; could not hear when spoken to in loud voice. 11.30 p.m., the same dose; no change in condition. 11.45 p.m., the same dose; stupor now fading away; delirium present; intolerant to light and noise; peculiar grin and cramp in face-muscles when attempting to talk; temp, 95.8; pulse very hard; intense thirst; less bleeding from punctures and blood thicker. 12 p.m., the same dose; no stupor now, but cramps in lower extremities;

no incoherency; only occasionally uneasy and senseless for a moment, and then rising suddenly like one startled when sound asleep. 12.30 a.m., no further symptoms; bleeding stopped; great thirst; eyes red and glaring; saccharine drinks given; no injection. 3 a.m., no sleep, but only slight slumber; no pain in foot; no bleeding; temperature, 98.8; thirst unabated; only drinks given.

Sept. 14th, 10 a.m.—Better, but talking slightly incoherent; received another injection of 1/12th grain of strychnine. 6 p.m., better; had good appetite; given milk and sago.

Sept. 15th, 6 a.m.—Better. 6 p.m.—Better; had three motions, rice and milk diet given, slept soundly between 10 a.m. and 2 p.m., no redness in eyes, swelling of foot abated.

Sept. 16th.—Better, only complaining of heaviness in head. At 9 p.m. had a fit of stupor all of a sudden, became insensible, and commenced to bleed again from the mucous membrane of mouth and nose. The patient became almost insensible, and could only be roused with difficulty. Twenty minims of liq. strychnine, equal to 1/6th grain, were now injected into the right arm.

At 9.20 stupor had passed away and consciousness was fully restored. From this time onward convalescence was uninterrupted, and patient was discharged cured on the 20th Sept., 1892.

In his remarks on this case Dr. Banerjee, after reporting that the snake with back broken in two places was brought to him on the following day from the exact locality where Rahimudden had been bitten, gives the following description of it:—Head, large and triangular; nostrils, large and kidney-shaped; scales, much imbricate, ventral scales 169, subcaudals 48; confluent, irregular ring-like, dark brown spots along the back, and with lateral black patches or rings with white borders. The head marking very peculiar double V shaped mark, the angle directed between the nostrils; interstitial coloration, yellowish brown, belly white, and with brown or amber spots; eyes, large, pupils erect, irides yellow; body, stout and compressed laterally; poison fangs, large and recurved, size about half an inch. The length of snake was 3 feet 5 inches, and from these characters it was identified to be the chain viper (*Duboia Russellii, Gray*), the most venomous of Indian vipers.

The total quantity of the antidote in this case administered was only 110 minims of a one in 120 solution of strychniæ acetas, or 11/12ths of a grain of that drug. Considering the extremely venomous nature of the snake and the large quantities of strychnine required in some of the previously reported cases of echis and bungarus bites, the quantity used seems disproportional, but this evidently is explained by the fact that only one of the fangs perforated deeply, and at the back of the foot, probably struck the bone before entering to its full length, the snake thus failing to impart the full quantity of venom at its disposal.

The chief interest of Dr. Banerjee's cases centres in the fact that they are mostly viper-bites. They prove conclusively, as do Feoktistow's experiments on the lower animals, that the theory of viper-poison being a blood poison, as asserted in all works on the subject, is not tenable and must be abandoned. If it effected changes in the blood, incompatible with life, strychnine, acting solely on the nerve-centres, could not possibly obliterate these changes within a few hours or even days. On the other hand the successful treatment of bungarus bite with strychnine places it beyond doubt that cobra-poison will also yield to it, if fearlessly and vigorously applied.

It is most gratifying to the writer to know from good authority that Sir Joseph Fayrer, the President of the Medical Board at the India office, has recommended to the English Government the adoption of the strychnine treatment of snakebite in India, and that this adoption will not be subject once more to the doubtful result of experiments on the lower animals, which, according to newspaper reports, were contemplated at Calcutta as a test. It would have been deplorable to see more precious time lost in these experiments, whilst the only proper subjects for experiments, the unfortunate natives, are perishing by thousands. The step taken by Sir Joseph Fayrer does honour both to his head and his heart, and if his recommendation is accepted and vigorously carried out it will still further increase the debt of gratitude which India owes to British rule, and with regard to its terrible snake plague, to the one Englishman who of all others has distinguished himself by an almost life long study of the subject and indefatigable labours for its alleviation.

Her Majesty the Queen has also been pleased most graciously to interest herself in this subject. Memorialised by the writer before Sir J. Fayrer's recommendation to the British Government, above alluded to, was known to him, our gracious Sovereign, ever intent on the welfare of her subjects, has resolved on having the writer's method thoroughly tried in India, and communicated this her intention to him in a despatch from the Secretary of State for the Colonies to His Excellency the Governor of Victoria, dated 11th Nov., 1892, inviting him, at the same time, to forward any proposals he may have to make direct to the Secretary to the Government of India in the Home Department; and thus adding one more to the many noble deeds that mark her benevolent, long, and glorious reign.

UNSUCCESSFUL CASES

Considering the newness of the strychnine treatment it would be folly to expect that the conditions necessary to insure success should have been observed in every case, and that every practitioner should at once have made himself familiar with it and the theory on which it is founded. Hence a few failures were unavoidable. Of these a record has been kept, but for obvious reasons the writer withholds it here. To give names and dates would be invidious, though the opponents of the treatment have exultingly pointed to the few deaths that have occurred as palpable proofs of its uselessness, some of them even going so far as to ascribe these deaths to the direct action of the antidote. There is, however, not a single case on record, in which death took place under strychnine-convulsions. All the patients died under palpable symptoms of snakebite-poisoning. As these symptoms have now been proven beyond all doubt to yield to strychnine, when properly administered, the inference that it was not so administered in the cases referred to becomes not only justifiable, but unavoidable. In one case only, that of a child of tender years, blood was vomited so copiously that death may be ascribed to that cause and the snake-poison combined, but in all the other six fatal ones, mostly of children, it was undoubtedly due to the snake-poison not being properly checked by the antidote. The gentlemen who officiated on these occasions were evidently not Banerjees, but the very reverse of their Indian confrère. They do not appear to have had very clear ideas of the absolute antagonism existing between the two poisons, and entirely disregarded the most important point in the treatment, namely, the necessity of administering the antidote until it has completely subdued the snake poison, regardless of the quantity that may be required for that purpose. In a few instances the treatment was correct enough at first, but when, as is often the case, a relapse took place after the patient had apparently recovered, the large quantity of the antidote already administered appears to have given rise to the erroneous notion that it would be useless to resort to it a second time, and thus, through this error and the fear of strychnine-convulsions, the patients were allowed to die. In most of the six fatal cases collected by the writer, however, the doses and total quantities given were altogether inadequate to cope with the poison. They did probably more harm than good, for the snake-poison when only partially checked by strychnine seems to renew its onslaught on the nerve-cells even more insidiously than when not interfered with at all. Convulsions also, as shown in cases, are sometimes called forth by this timid use of the antidote.

A few instances will show the correctness of these observations. Thus an old woman sleeping in a shed is awakened at daylight by a tiger snake having fastened on to her wrist. She pulls off the snake, alarms the neighbours, and a doctor, living only a mile away from the place, is sent for. He appears on the scene four hours afterwards, when complete coma and collapse has set in, makes two injections of gr. 1/15 each, which of course had no effect and the patient is allowed to die without any further effort on the part of her medical attendant. Case 2.—A boy of 10 years is admitted to a N. S. Wales hospital in a state of complete collapse, barely alive, having been bitten by a brown snake 22 hours before admission. Instead of a rousing injection of at least 15 minims and the same or smaller ones repeated at short intervals, he receives only 5 minims of liq. strychniæ P.B. every twenty minutes, when death was imminent, and dies 65 minutes after admission. Case 3 is also that of a boy in an hospital. He is admitted fully conscious and apparently but slightly under the influence of snake-poison, for a five minims injection is reported to have removed the symptoms. On the following day, however, he became comatose, and instead of having the antidote freely administered, gets only one more injection of five minims and dies in coma. Case 4 is even worse. A little girl of 3 years, bitten by a tiger snake, receives three minim injections every half-hour, and after three of them, whilst in a state of complete coma, gets convulsions. These are attributed to the strychnine, which thereupon is withheld, the finale being death in coma.

There can be no doubt that in all these cases life could have been preserved under a more energetic treatment. Hereafter, when theory and treatment are better understood, and when officialdom has seen fit to issue instructions as to the proper treatment of snakebite to medical practitioners, such cases as those cited will be put down as malpractice and have to be accounted for. Until then the guardians of the health and the lives of her Majesty's subjects, and a certain portion of the medical press of Australia, superciliously and persistently ignoring the subject, are more responsible for the lives lost than the busy country practitioner, who may not have had time or opportunity to inform himself thoroughly on a comparatively new subject, more especially at a period when Banerjee had not yet taught us that in administering strychnine as antidote to snake-poison we can venture into grains of it with impunity.

Since the above chapters were put in proof, the writer has seen a fatal case of tiger snake bite, conveying two lessons of such interest and importance that it must be placed on record here. It illustrates in an extraordinary and forcible degree the erratic, capricious, and insidious course the snake-poison takes at times.

A handsome girl of 17 is bitten in a bathroom on the back of the second right toe at dusk on a Sunday evening by a half-grown tiger snake, subsequently caught and killed in the room. She does not suspect snakebite, and no ligature is applied until the poison has been absorbed and overpowers her. Instead of sinking into coma, she becomes unconscious for a short time only. Her brain then clears itself, and all symptoms seem to disappear so completely that when a medical man of undoubted ability and skill sees her a few hours after the bite, she declares herself quite well again, and does not appear to require any treatment, least of all that by strychnine injections. She passes a good night, but on Monday morning symptoms denoting paresis of the respiratory and glosso-pharyngeal centres make their appearance, almost identical with those described by Indian writers as following cobra-bite. She has difficulty in breathing and swallowing, but one injection of 1/10th of a grain removes it completely and speedily, and once more all danger is thought to be past. On Monday evening, however, dyspnœa and dysphagia appear again in an aggravated form. The urine also becomes scanty and loaded with albuminates. Strychnine now is again resorted to, but it fails to act as before, and from hour to hour the young lady's condition becomes more critical. When the writer reached her on Tuesday afternoon, 42 hours after the bite, paralysis of the centres named was imminent, and her case appeared a hopeless one, unless a vigorous use of strychnine yet turned the scales in her favour. One-tenth grain doses were therefore injected every half-hour, and continued until the physiological action of the drug showed itself. This took place, but failed to have the least effect on the affected centres; and complete paralysis ensued 45 hours after the infliction of the fatal bite.

The first lesson the Australian practitioner should learn from this sad case is that of extreme care and caution in dealing with any case of snakebite, no matter how slight it may appear at first sight. It is not for the first time we have been taught this lesson, though it has rarely, if ever, been conveyed in so singular a manner. Recent utterances about the innocuousness of Australian snake-poison find a fitting answer in this melancholy occurrence.

The second lesson it conveys is a new one, even to the writer. From the fact of one strychnine injection removing all poison-symptoms early on Monday, but the free use of the antidote failing entirely to have this effect on Monday night and on Tuesday, we are warranted to draw the conclusion that the antidote can only be relied on within the first 24 hours after the bite; and that, after this period, the snake-poison produces organic changes in the affected nerve-cells, preventing their depressed functional activity from being restored by the antidote. Further observations, of course, are required to confirm these conclusions. Their correctness, however, appears to be borne out by the fact observed by the writer, that the larger domestic animals, who sometimes linger on for days after being bitten by a snake, usually recover under the strychnine treatment if it is applied immediately or soon after a bite, but die when found and treated in an advanced stage of the malady.

That the grave kidney complication, checking the elimination of the poison from the system, militated against recovery in this case, and greatly influenced the singular course of the poisoning process, cannot be doubted.

CONCLUSION

In the little work submitted herewith to the medical profession and the general public, for both of whom it is intended, the author may justly claim to have solved the difficult and long-standing problem of snake-poison. We have at last a correct theory of its action, and, what is of more importance to the public, we have an effective antidote. These facts, being as fully established in these pages as any scientific facts can be, the most exacting and even captious criticism will not upset, nor can further research add anything very material to the writer's deductions and their final result.

In order to show how an obscure Australian country practitioner succeeded in a discovery, for which all his predecessors in this field of research had laboured in vain, it will be necessary in conclusion to give a short history of the discovery as by slow degrees it has originated and matured in the writer's mind, who during the last 35 years with respect to this subject had followed the advice which Schiller gives in his grand poem, "Die Glocke:" —

> Wer etwas Treffliches leisten will,
> Hätt' gern was Grossesgeboren,
> Der sammle still und unerschlafft
> Im kleinsten Punkte die grösste Kraft,

which, translated into English, means that whoever aims at any great achievement must quietly, but indefatigably, concentrate the highest force on the smallest point. Now this smallest point has to the writer been snake-poison from the very commencement of his Australian career. When yet a new-chum, a vigorous tiger snake gave him the first lesson on the action of the insidious venom which nearly cost him his life, but afforded some valuable glimpses into the mystery of snakebite—in fact, gave him the key to unlock that mystery. On analysing the horrid sensations he had experienced before he lost consciousness, and even after regaining it, he saw "depressed nerve-action, emanating from the central nervous system," written on the face of every one of them, so much so that this became the foundation and corner stone of his present structure, which, however, it took him a quarter of a century to erect; for the material he required, namely, cases of snakebite observed from an early stage, and from which all disturbing elements were excluded, did not occur very frequently in his practice. Though he lived all the time among mountains, the beautiful Australian Alps, on the rivers and creeks of which snakes are abundant, and though these creatures and anything connected with them had an almost fascinating interest for him, years sometimes elapsed without adding one single good case to his notes. Sometimes his patients were dead when he reached them, and all his entreaties for an autopsy were in vain with the relatives. More frequently he found that they were not bitten at all, and only suffered from the effects of fear or of enormous doses of alcohol. On persons really bitten, but completely paralysed and comatose, observations were also unsatisfactory, as they had to be supplemented by second-hand evidence obtained from those who had been with them before they became unconscious. Thus within 25 years the author did not see more than half-a-dozen really instructive cases; and frequently his desire for more evidence overcame his reluctance to inflict on animals the agony of snakebite he had himself endured, and he made a few experiments, but soon gave them up again as unsatisfactory. All the evidence, however, he had thus far collected tended to confirm the correctness of his ideas as to the action of snake-poison. At last, some ten years ago, he obtained absolute certainty, and this, strange to relate, by a case of spider bite.

He was called early one morning to visit a little boy, two years old, and on examination found that he presented symptoms almost identical with those of snakebite poisoning. Although there was no evidence of the child having come in contact with a snake, the writer naturally concluded that during the night a snake had obtained access to the bedroom through the open door or window, and after biting the child sleeping in its low cot, had escaped again. He therefore searched most carefully for the usual two punctures, but they were not to be found. The child evidently laboured under the effect of some poison, and spiderbite suggested itself, but the symptoms were so much more aggravated than anything the writer had frequently seen of spiderbite that he hesitated to accept it as the cause, although it appeared almost the only possible one. A careful inquiry into the history of the case elicited from the mother the important fact that on the previous afternoon the little fellow, just able to toddle about, had gradually lost the use of his legs, and also become very peevish, and that suspecting nothing but a little temporary indisposition, she had put him to bed, to find him in the morning all but dead. He was scarcely breathing when the writer saw him, and only the stethoscope gave evidence of the heart still beating feebly. His body was very cold, pupils widely dilated, and the sight even apparently gone, the eyes wide open, staring fixedly upwards and not noticing a lighted match in closest proximity to them. Consciousness also appeared extinct, as liquids introduced into the mouth were not swallowed. Examining once more for traces of spiderbite in the skin, the writer noticed faint red stripes extending up the arm from a little cut on the right index finger near the nail, and on inquiry it was ascertained at last from an elder brother that he had seen the child pick up a little black spider with a red back, hold it for some time between thumb and index finger, and then throw it away. This was evidently the Katipo (*Latrodectus icelio*), the poison of which acts on the same principle as snake-poison, but generally much milder. The greater severity of its action in this case was accounted for by the mandibles having been inserted into the cut, and the insect, being squeezed by the child, having emptied the whole available contents of its poison gland into the cellular tissue exposed in the cut, whence it was quickly absorbed. This also accounted for the absence of all irritation and of the neuralgic pains usually accompanying spiderbite, when the mandibles merely perforate the epidermis and the poison is deposited in the upper cutis, where absorption is slow and local irritation consequently greater.

Minuteness of detail in relating this case must be excused on account of the extreme interest and importance attached to it. Being brought about under such peculiar and almost unique circumstances it presented the effects of spider-poison in a superlative degree and showed them to be identical with those of snake-poison. But whilst the latter ushers in the symptoms with such rapidity that they cover each other and are difficult of separate analysis, in this case the highly significant paresis of the lower extremities, evidently of central origin, remained separate for some time. Taking this symptom for his guide and interpreting the formidable array of the others, developed during the night, on the same principle, the writer's diagnosis of the case, as it presented itself to him, was paralysis of the motor and vaso-motor nerve-centres. This, he found, and this alone could explain all the symptoms, and he therefore determined to put its correctness to a practical test. There was but one remedy to make this test with and this had to be applied without delay, for the child was rapidly sinking and had almost ceased to breathe. *One twelfth of a grain* of strychnine was therefore injected in the arm, a bold dose for so young a child, but, as the result showed, exactly the one that was required. The test was eminently successful. Having to leave the child immediately after the injection, the writer on returning in half an hour found his little patient sitting up in bed, perfectly restored, with both poisons so completely neutralising each other, that not a trace of either could be detected. Thus the writer's structure was at last completed, and an insignificant spider furnished the last material required for an important discovery.

There are a few hypothetical points yet in the explanation of some of the symptoms of snakebite-poisoning by the writer's theory, but these imperfections are more those of science than of the theory. The whole subject of vaso-motor paralysis for instance, and of the pathological changes that follow it, is more or less a *terra incognita*. Diapedesis is now supposed to be the result of blood pressure, but it occurs in snakebite, where blood pressure is at zero. Feoktistow, we have seen, produced it locally on the mesentery of animals with normal blood pressure, whilst Banerjee arrested by strychnine-injections profuse hæmorrhages from all the mucous surfaces, which were no doubt the result of diapedesis. We know that neither snake-poison nor strychnine affect the nerve ends but only the nerve cells. There must therefore be nerve cells at or near the terminations of the nerves regulating the capillary circulation in the mucous membranes, but microscopical anatomy has yet to find them, for minute ganglia have only been discovered at present in sympathetic nerve ends of the abdomen.

On other subjects also, besides that of vaso-motor paralysis, the strychnine treatment of snakebite has thrown an unexpected light. We did not know before it was demonstrated by this treatment that sleep is merely a reduced discharge of motor-nerve force, a partial turning off of the motor-batteries, by which, through rest, they are invigorated for fresh action during the waking hours, and that the degrees of this reduction range in their effects from sleep, more or less deep, down to coma, and can be raised again from coma to sleep, and from sleep to complete wakefulness. We knew that every movement and action is brought about by a discharge of this force, but we did not know that even the silent thought must be carried on the wings of it, and cannot take place without it, at least not in our present state of existence. All these important revelations are now the property of science, and it will be well for science to take note of them.

In conclusion, the writer may be permitted to express his joy and thankfulness for having been made the instrument, by Divine Providence, to confer a boon on humanity that will prevent much suffering and thousands of premature, untimely deaths.